DRUGS AND ATHLETIC PERFORMANCE

DRUGS AND ATHLETIC PERFORMANCE

By

MELVIN H. WILLIAMS, Ph.D.

Director
Human Performance Laboratory
Old Dominion University
Norfolk, Virginia

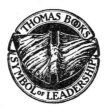

CHARLES C THOMAS • **PUBLISHER**
Springfield • Illinois • U.S.A.

749789
DLC

11-25-81JH

Published and Distributed Throughout the World by
CHARLES C THOMAS • PUBLISHER
Bannerstone House
301-327 East Lawrence Avenue, Springfield, Illinois, U.S.A.

With THOMAS BOOKS *careful attention is given to all details of
manufacturing and design. It is the Publisher's desire to present books
that are satisfactory as to their physical qualities and artistic possibilities
and appropriate for their particular use.* THOMAS BOOKS *will be true
to those laws of quality that assure a good name and good will.*

Printed in the United States of America
W-2

Library of Congress Cataloging in Publication Data

Williams, Melvin H
    Drugs and athletic performance.

    Bibliography: p.
    1. Doping in sports. I. Title.
[DNLM: 1. Drug abuse. 2. Ethics. 3. Sport,
Medicine. QT260 W727d 1974]
RC1230.W54   615.7   73-19709
ISBN 0-398-03064-2

To my mother and late father,
who epitomize the terms Mom and Dad

PREFACE

As ONE OF THE basic characteristics of man is to play, it was only a matter of time, given the nature of man for organization and the advent of increased leisure time, until play activities developed into a more serious sphere of life, i.e. sports. Although sports, or some type of organized play, has been an integral part of most cultures from antiquity, it was not until this century, particularly within the past two decades, that sports participation and the sports industry experienced such phenomenal growth. In order to perceive the impact of sport on American culture one need only consider the coverage devoted to athletics in radio, television, newspapers and magazines; the sporting goods industry is a multi-billion dollar business, while the seal of approval of the NFL, NHL, ABA, or NBA is eagerly pursued by manufacturers of diverse products in order to enhance their sales appeal. Similar practices are evident in other countries around the world.

Why man engages in sport is a philosophical question which has been the subject of several treatises, notably *Homo Ludens* by Johan Huizinga. Considering the value which society assigns to sport, it is only natural that man participates in such activity in an attempt to achieve self-actualization. Idealistically, sport provides an excellent opportunity for man to actualize his physical potential, whether in competition with himself or others. A little more realistically, the basic objective of sport is to win—to score more points, to jump higher, run faster, throw farther—to be victorious against your opponent or excel previously established records. However, in order to be acceptable, the athlete's endeavors must be within the established rules and guidelines for his particular sport—which brings us to the muddled concept of sports ethics.

Ethics, according to Webster, involves the study of ideal

human character, actions and ends. When applied to a particular controversial situation, the questioned behavior is either right or wrong, ethical or unethical, moral or immoral, a decision which may be dependent upon the individual's interpretation of what constitutes "ideal human character." Sports represent a sphere of life whereby the ordinary rules and ethics of organized civilization may be suspended. For example, it may be wrong to attempt to physically abuse your fellow man in everyday life situations, but evidence the basic objectives of the boxer or the defensive lineman in football. What is ethical in sport is, to say the least, an extremely complex question. One can think of numerous instances in the administration and conduct of sports where the questions of ethics may be raised; the use of various drugs is one of the major ethical problems which confronts administrators of amateur athletic governing organizations. The physician for the professional team who prescribes amphetamines and anabolic steroids may be applauded by the coaches and management, but his actions may be appalling to some of his medical colleagues.

Most athletic governing bodies have rules proscribing the use of certain drugs in athletic competition. Basically, the deciding factor is whether or not the drug is therapeutic in nature. But what is therapeutic? If aspirin is utilized to relieve a headache and concomitantly increases the threshold level for pain during an athletic event, is it still therapeutic or has it crossed the gray line into illegality? How many cups of coffee, with each cup containing a therapeutic dose of caffeine, are construed as an attempt to enhance performance through drugs? Acetylsalicylic acid and caffeine are not banned, but they do produce effects on the CNS which may be beneficial to the athlete. And what of substances which are proscribed by the rules? If a sympathomimetic is prescribed as medication by a physician, should the athlete be barred from competition? If an athlete is injured in competing, may he receive pain pills in order to continue? The decision to utilize these substances rests in the ethical judgment of the athlete's physician. However, their use under current regulations of several athletic governing bodies may constitute grounds for elimination from competition.

What problems face the athlete and the rules-formulating bodies in the future. Platt (403), discussing the scientific urgencies of the next ten years, indicated that we are moving into the era of supermedicine, while Toffler, in his best-seller *Future Shock*, noted that by the year 2000, or sooner, personality altering drugs may be commonly used. If a medicine can be produced which will increase man's performance, and yet have no adverse side effects, should it be illegal to use it if available to all? Even more grandiose plans for increasing athletic performance may be forthcoming. According to Heywood Hale Broun (67), certain countries are already evaluating a child's physical and athletic ability upon entrance into school, usually at five years of age, and directing the individual to his most suitable sport. Those who excel are placed into special schools for advanced training and special diets, which may include drug therapy. Is it only a matter of time until this concept is applied to the pre-natal stage. Euphenics, or the engineering of human development, is in an embryonic stage, but as scientists continue to unravel the intricacies of human embryology, the day of gene manipulation and development of the superhuman, or superathlete, draws closer and closer.

The purpose of this preface is not to debate or in any way attempt to resolve ethical issues concerned with the use of drugs in sport, but simply to raise questions relative to current and future status. The problems of drug use in contemporary athletics are many and complex, and may become even more involved in the future. If sound guidelines are to be developed by athletic governing bodies, extensive research needs to be conducted in order to provide the facts relative to the establishment of such guidelines. This book is an attempt to synthesize the specific research which has been conducted up to the present concerning the effect of various drugs on athletic performance. Athletic performance, for the purpose of this book, is interpreted broadly and includes all those physiological and psychological parameters which may be important contributing factors to athletic success.

A number of individuals have been most helpful during the developmental stages of this book. I would especially like to thank the staff of the National Library of Medicine for their gracious cooperation during the literature search. Much appreciation is due Guenther and Mary Ann Dietz for their assistance in the translation of German and French reports.

M.H.W.

CONTENTS

		Page
Preface	....	vii

Chapter
1	INTRODUCTION TO THE DRUG PROBLEM IN ATHLETICS	3
2	DRUGS AFFECTING THE NERVOUS SYSTEM—STIMULANTS	20
3	DRUGS AFFECTING THE NERVOUS SYSTEM—DEPRESSANTS	61
4	DRUGS AFFECTING THE MUSCULAR SYSTEM	87
5	DRUGS AFFECTING THE CARDIOVASCULAR SYSTEM	109
6	RESEARCH AND THE DOPING PROBLEM	130

Bibliography	....	137
Glossary	....	169
Author Index	....	183
Subject Index	....	189

DRUGS AND ATHLETIC PERFORMANCE

CHAPTER 1

INTRODUCTION TO THE DRUG PROBLEM IN ATHLETICS

Although drugs, in one form or another, have been with mankind since antiquity, it was not until the last one hundred years that the pharmacological industry has undergone such tremendous growth. According to Ray (416), the development of vaccines, broad-spectrum antibiotics, and tranquilizers has characterized three recent major drug revolutions.

The fourth pharmacological revolution is still in the developmental stage, and the impact upon society may be greater than the other three combined. The increasing emphasis on pleasure tends to draw individuals to the drug culture; while in the past drugs were utilized primarily for sick individuals, the time has arrived when healthy individuals are using variant drugs for their effect in altering personality or increasing social interaction. Thus we are entering the era of biological engineering, where drugs and even surgical techniques may be utilized to control developmental stages of man's mind and body. Indeed, Toffler, in his best-seller *Future Shock*, hypothesized that an entire industry will be developed around the merchandising of pleasure through drugs, and it may not be uncommon to start the day with orange juice laced with amphetamines.

As Western civilization has been successful in creating a number of *instant devices* there is a growing tendency for our society to want instant pleasure, such as can be elicited from certain drugs. As this attitude may permeate society in general,

3

it may carry over into the sports world and possibly influence the athlete's decision to utilize drugs for instant success.

ERGOGENIC AIDS

Translated literally, the term ergogenic means tending to increase work, or work producing. Thus, any treatment which could produce ergogenic effects in man might prove to be beneficial in sports for it might increase his physical or mental capacity. Athletes have utilized a variety of mechanical, pharmacological and nutritional substances, supposedly ergogenic in nature, in an effort to increase performance capacity. Listed below are a number of substances or treatments which have been used over the years, several of which are still in prominent use today:

Alcohol
Alkalies
Amphetamines and other sympathomimetic drugs
Anabolic Steroids
Aspartates
Caffeine
Cardiovascular stimulants
Cold applications
Glucose preparations
Heat applications
Hormones
Hypnosis
Information feedback
Lecithin
Massage
Mental practice
Negatively ionized air
Oxygen
Peripheral vasodilators
Protein supplements
Sodium chloride

Ultraviolet rays
Vitamin and mineral supplements
Wheat germ oil

Due to the diverse nature of these substances, or treatments, there are varied hypotheses which account for the beneficial effects they are alleged to produce. The rationale for their use may be reduced to two categories: (a) the substances may directly influence the physiological capacity of a particular body system which contributes to the athletic performance, or (b) the substance may remove psychological restraints which may limit physiological capacity. An example of the first category would be the application of heat in order to increase the circulation to a particular part of the body, while hypnosis would represent a treatment falling into the second category. Certain substances, such as pharmacological agents, may be placed into both categories as they exert concomitant physiological and psychological effects upon the performer.

Although authorities such as Fowler (177) and Cooper (108) argue that ergogenic aids have no significant beneficial effect upon physical performance, many athletes contend that certain substances give them that "winning edge" necessary in championship performance. Consider the differences in the gold medal and silver medal times in Olympic competion. With timers accurate to thousandths of a second, just a minute physiological or psychological advantage may determine which national anthem is played when the medalists take to the award platform. Indeed, research has been conducted to determine that penicillin and other therapeutic drugs will not adversely affect an athlete's performance (195, 378).

There appears to be little debate or controversy over some ergogenic aids, while a great deal of deliberation centers around others. In the contemporary amateur athletic society, the acceptance spectrum of ergogenic aids runs the gamut from permissive use of massage to rather universal disapproval of certain classes of drugs. An excellent treatise on ergogenic aids in general has been edited by Morgan (360), with reports that such benign substances as carbohydrates, cold water applications, water and electrolyte replacement, mental practice and information feedback may be ergogenic under specific conditions. Vanek and Cratty (517) report that an autogenic technique, or the induction of self-hypnosis, may also be beneficial. Thus, while in the past the term ergogenic has had a negative connotation in the eyes of the athletic rules makers, there are certain phenomena or techniques which may influence performance positively and possibly should be incorporated into the training and education regimen of the athlete.

On the other hand, there are a variety of substances, primarily pharmacological in nature, which for legal, ethical or medical rationale are deemed unacceptable for use in association with athletic contests. Most individuals are aware of the contemporary drug scene in the American society. In the sport society, the wide use of drugs as ergogenic aids in recent years has prompted athletic governing bodies to legislate and educate against their use. Concern has even reached the federal government level, as in 1973 a House Special Education Committee under the direction of James G. O'Hara, D-Michigan, investigated whether college athletes were being exposed to the drug culture as part of the victory syndrome (424).

The negative connotation of ergogenic aids is directed primarily towards the pharmacological agents, for they raise the legal, ethical and medical controversies. Consequently, they are the substances which should receive considerable research attention in order to determine their effectiveness or ineffectiveness in the athletic arena.

DRUGS IN ATHLETICS—DOPING

The use of drugs to enhance athletic performance is not the domain of modern civilized society, as certain substances were used in antiquity and throughout the years in order to increase work capacity. Csaky (120) noted that the first recorded incidence of doping was in the Garden of Eden when Adam and Eve believed the apple would give them God-like powers. Ancient Greeks ate sesame seeds, the legendary Berserkers in Norwegian mythology used bufotein, while the Andean Indians and Australian aborigines chewed, respectively, coca leaves and the pituri plant for stimulating and antifatiguing effects. Catton, in his classic Civil War account, indicated the *Army of the Potomac* maintained its energy due to the tremendous amount of coffee the soldiers consumed. From the early part of this century, boxers, marathon runners, European cyclists, baseball and soccer players, Olympic contestants and other athletes have used numerous pharmaceutical agents as ergogenic aids. As an example, Tatarelli (499) experimented with a compound called Nike, consisting of vitamin C, glucose, potassium acid tartrate, kola, and phosphorilamine, in a study concerning the pharmaco-biological potentiation of the athlete. However, it is only in recent years that drug use in athletics has received considerable attention, probably because of the national and international drug problem as a whole.

Prevalence

Although the abuse of drugs in sports may appear to be greatest on the collegiate and professional levels, recent evidence has revealed increasing usage on the high school level. Although Smith (483) reported little drug use in athletes in a brief local community survey, Baugh (46), in a report to the American School Health Association, indicated that 10 per cent of the male and female athletes involved in his survey had used stimulant-type drugs while participating in an athletic event. Irwin (267) also discussed reports of the wide-spread use of drugs, particularly amphetamines, in the high school athletic arena, indicating the use has filtered down to athletes at the age of fourteen and fifteen. Irwin also indicated drug use is prominent among college athletes. A thorough report should be forthcoming next year, as the National Collegiate Athletic Association (NCAA) is currently conducting a nationwide survey of drug use in collegiate athletics. On the professional level, Jim Bouton, in his book *Ball Four,* hypothesized that approximately 40 percent of major league players used bennies (amphetamine) or greenies (a combination of amphetamines and barbiturates) in order to enhance performance. A number of professional football players have been on steroids for years in an attempt to increase body mass, and personal conversations with several NFL and CFL players have also revealed widespread use of amphetamines and pain killers in that sport. Further documentation of the prevalence of drugs in sports is offered by Gilbert in a three part analysis (202, 203, 204).

Discussing the universality of sport, Mollet (359) indicated that athletes are used as ambassadors, with a victory in sport being regarded as a victory for the country, and possibly extrapolated to include the political or economic system of that country. Thus, the prevalence of drug use in athletics is not only a national, but an international problem, and has been the subject of several international sports medicine symposia in the past ten years. The primary concerns at these meetings have been the definition of doping and the development of effective legislation designed to prevent its use in sports.

Definition

In order to effectively legislate against doping, first the term has to be explicitly defined. In 1939, Boje (56) indicated the term doping was used in a general sense to describe any method of temporarily improving athletic performance, either during training or in connection with competition. He included not only drugs such as Benzedrine®, cocaine or caffeine, but also other aids such as glucose, vitamins, oxygen inhalation, massage and even cheering. Although Boje noted that doping was a serious question at that time, he gave no indication of legislation against it. Following the Rome Olympics in 1960, increased international attention was devoted to doping. Venerando (518), in agreement with Boje, stated that doping is not necessarily restricted to a medicament or drug, but any system or practice which aims to artificially increase the physiological efficiency of man or animal. In a restrictive sense, however, he did note that doping can be considered within the limits of pharmacology. Thus, doping today is usually associated with pharmacological potentiation of athletic power, but the interpretation of just what exactly constitutes pharmacological doping is another matter.

The various athletic governing bodies proscribe the use of a variety of drugs in sports. The National Federation of State High School Athletic Associations' rules state that whether done unknowingly, tacitly, secretly, or openly, the use of unwarranted ergogenic aids in sports is unequivocally condemned, i.e. drugs used to increase body capacity by eliminating fatigue symptoms (297). In a brief description, the NCAA indicated that the use of nontherapeutic drugs is not in keeping with the aims and purposes of amateur athletics and is prohibited. Both the International Amateur Athletic Federation (IAAF) and the International Olympic Committee (IOC) elaborate on the definition of doping. Rule 144 of the IAAF represents anti-doping legislation on the international scene. In general, the rule prohibits the use by or distribution to a competitor of those substances which could have the effect of improving artificially the competitor's physical and/or mental condition and so augmenting his athletic performance. It is forbidden before or during competition. Specific drugs include:

(a) *Psychomotor stimulant drugs*

amphetamine	methylphenidate
benzphetamine	norpseudo ephedrine
cocaine	pemoline
diethylpropion	phendimetrazine
dimethylamphetamine	phenmetrazine
ethylamphetamine	phentermine
fencamfamin	pipradol
fenproporex	prolintane
methylamphetamine	and related compounds

(b) *Sympathomimetic amines*

ephedrine	
methylephedrine	
methoxyphenamine	and related compounds

(c) *Miscellaneous central nervous system stimulants*

amiphenazole	nikethamide
bemegride	strychnine
leptazole	and related compounds

(d) *Narcotic analgesics*

morphine	pethidine	
heroin	dextromoramide	
methadone	dipipanone	and related compounds

(e) Anabolic steroids

As indicated by the IAAF, the list is not comprehensive. In essence, any substance which may be used to increase performance is prohibited.

The Medical Commission of the IOC defines doping as follows:

> Doping is the administration of or the use by a competing athlete of any substance foreign to the body or of any physiological substance taken in abnormal quantity or taken by an abnormal route of entry into the body, with the sole intention of increasing in an artificial and unfair manner his performance in competition. When necessity demands medical treatment with any substance which because of its nature, dosage, or application is able to boost the athlete's performance in competition in an artificial and unfair manner, this is to be regarded as doping.

Drugs specifically proscribed by the IOC included adrenalin, amphetamines and related compounds, CNS stimulants, ethyl alcohol, narcotics such as morphine, cardiovascular drugs, vasodilators, tranquilizers, antidepressants, muscular relaxants, and anabolic or androgenic hormones (309). However, Fischbach (165) recently noted that alcohol and anabolic steroids were not specifically mentioned on the IOC list for the 1972 Munich Olympics.

The final sentence of the IOC definition above has been the subject of debate. There would appear to be legitimate uses for some drugs in athletics, e.g. to lessen pain of athletic injuries, to relieve muscle spasms, to cure headaches, dysmenorrhea and a variety of other conditions which might hamper an athlete's normal performance. In the 1972 Munich Olympics, an American swimmer, Rick DeMont, was deprived of an earned gold medal, because as an asthmatic he was receiving medicine which contained ephedrine, a sympathomimetic drug. The problem is—where does therapy end and doping begin?

In 1965, Fishbach (163) stated that the classical doping agents should be prohibited, namely the stimulants and narcotics, but that sports pharmaca which, at normal dosage, have a physiological but nontoxic action should be permitted under sportsmedical control. This group would include sedatives, soporifics, certain analgesics, and some substances from the analeptic series. In a more recent publication by the American Association for Health, Physical Education and Recreation (2), the definition of doping has been restricted to the use of prescription drugs for other than clinically justified purposes. This definition would not take into consideration such purported aids as alcohol, blood doping, over-the-counter drugs, or caffeine—even though the authors indicated that caffeine is becoming increasingly popular as a stimulant in athletics.

Undoubtedly no one definition of doping would satisfy all individuals or all athletic governing bodies. As an example, the International Cycling Union allows ephedrine, whereas the IOC does not (462). Indeed, Porritt (408) indicated that the definition of doping is, if not impossible, at least extremely difficult. However, he noted that those individuals involved in sport know exactly what it means, and that the definition lies not in words, but in integrity of character.

Detection

Engaging in prophecy, Lees (321) noted in 1949 that:

a time may come when people take Benzedrine in a suitably flavored drink for breakfast. . . . One day we may have to test students for benzedrine before exams, the way we test race horses. It is doubtful that benzedrine will ever be considered good form on the race track or in athletic events, but a time may come when, like liquor, it will be quite all right socially if you carry it like a gentleman.

Twenty-five years later, part of his statement holds true—drugs are banned in athletic events involving both humans and animals. Drug abuse in horse racing was extremely prevalent in the 1930's when, according to Clarke (99), over half of the horses running were said to be doped. In a review of the literature, he noted over eighty different compounds had been detected in an attempt to improve or deter performance. One of the compounds used during the thirties contained 1½ grams of heroin, 2½ grams of strychnine, 2 minims of nitroglycerin, 5 minims of digitalis, and 2 ounces of cola nut (257). The development of accurate detection methods was effective in controlling the problem, and in the 1951 to 1967 period, only a minute percentage of horses were detected as having been doped. Clarke indicated, however, that there are still problems in detecting drugs in race horses as there are numerous drugs available and the screening techniques can only detect a limited number. For the interested reader, Schubert (451) presents a detailed discussion of doping horses with particular emphasis to identification and metabolism of some common drugs used to dope horses. He periodically extrapolates the possible application to the problem of drugs in human athletes. Needless to say, although the use of detection techniques in horse racing has rather successfully curtailed drug abuse, there are special problems associated with testing humans.

Prokop (412 ,413) and Venerando (518) discussed the problems facing contemporary athletic governing bodies in their attempt to promote effective international anti-doping legislation. As was indicated previously in this text, most major associations have banned doping. However, the legislation, in order to be effective, has to be enforced; the legal, technical and organizational details of drug detection have posed numerous problems.

The scientific techniques for detecting certain drugs in humans are available. Drugs are distributed throughout the body water; therefore, analyses of sweat, saliva, urine or blood have been used for detection purposes. Since the amphetamines and its congeners appear to be the most abused drugs in athletics, various techniques have been developed for their detection in biological fluids. Urine is the preferred medium, and the most common procedure involves chromatography. In the late 1950's and early 1960's, the paper chromatographic technique was the main detection method used to determine the presence of amphetamine in the urine. More recent techniques include combinations of thin-layer chromatography (TLC), gas-liquid chromatography (GLC), mass spectroscopy (MS) or micro-infrared spectroscopy (MIS). Venerando (518) discussed the historical aspects involving detection methods, while detailed information concerning different detection procedures were described by Beckett and his colleagues (48), Cartoni and Cavalli (87), and Moerman and de Vleeschhouwer (358). Combination methods are usually used since Marozzi (344) indicated that many substances containing at least one amine group, although of very different pharmacological activity, may be confused with amphetamine on the basis of the Vidic test if it was not applied in conjunction with another completely different test. Although the technical procedures vary slightly between the different methods available for the detection of amphetamines and its congeners, the basic procedure involves an extraction process with ether, a screening technique with either TLC or GLC, and a follow-up of suspicious samples by either GLC, MS, or MIS. The process is effective 1 to 2 hours after ingestion until 3 to 4 days later. Detection techniques such as the above have been effectively employed in Olympic and other international athletic competition (354).

Although the scientific expertise is available for detecting amphetamines and its congeners, there are other unsolved problems associated with drug detection. First, the tests developed are primarily aimed at the amphetamine group. Different tests would need to be employed for the other proscribed drugs such as alcohol, analgesics, tranquilizers, vasodilators, cardiovascular drugs or anabolic steroids. In the case of steroids, the possibilities of detecting their use is limited, since they are not used in conjunction with the actual competitive event, but in the training period prior to competition. Moreover, R. W. Pritchard, chairman of the NCAA Drug Education Committee, noted they are still looking for a complete list of drugs to be banned before the NCAA implements detection methods (376). Secondly, the expenses involved in the organizational details and the chromatographic procedures may be prohibitive. A recent article (376) indicated lack of financing may prevent drug detection enforcement at NCAA championship events. Lastly, the legality of the detection procedures is being questioned. Pritchard (376) reported legal red tape is another hurdle to implementation of a drug detection program for NCAA championship events, while the NFL Players Association is against detection methods, based upon the legal aspects surrounding invasion of privacy.

Thus, while most athletic governing bodies have developed a detailed procedure involving the collection, registration, storage and analysis of urine, primarily for the amphetamine-like substances, there are still difficulties concerning the identification of other compounds as well as economic and legal ramifications. The procedure may be appropriate for high-level international competition, but at the present time is not feasible for most other athletic events.

The Paradox of Doping

The rationale against doping basically revolves around two issues: (a) medical reasons due to the potential pharmacotoxic dangers of certain drugs, and (b) sport ethics. The first reason is justification enough; however, statements regarding sport ethics and doping are usually paradoxical.

From a neuropsychiatric viewpoint, Roubicek (438) indicated that the main problems with the use of doping agents in sports are the pharmacotoxic effects of overdoses in an acute attempt to enhance performance with centrally acting substances, and the psychotoxic effects of habit formation due to chronic use of certain drugs. The literature is replete with incidents involving drug dangers in athletics. Murphy (364) noted the death of two Danish bicyclists during the 1960 Rome Olympics due to use of a potent vasodilator. Amphetamines have been implicated in the deaths of bicyclists (101) and a French Olympic basketball player in the 1968 games at Mexico City (364). In 1972, Pawlucki (398) indicated, according to unofficial data, that approximately 70 cases of death have occurred in the last few years due to doping in athletics. Thus, although a definite cause and effect relationship has not been established between the use of drugs, such as amphetamine, and deaths in athletics, it would appear prudent to proscribe their use based on the information at hand. The effect amphetamine may have in delaying subjective symptoms of fatigue, in combination with a high environmental heat stress index, may predispose the athlete to heat stroke. The popularity of anabolic steroids may predispose the athlete to several health problems, which are discussed in more detail in Chapter 4. The case against doping, based upon definite health hazards, appears to be logically constructed.

On the other hand, the sports ethic rationale against doping appears to be a paradox. Since athletic competition is designed to be a comparison of man's innate and self-developed ability, the utilization of drugs to enhance performance is considered unethical (100, 368). Indeed, a national conference on value in sports reported the use of any drug to improve athletic performance is unethical in the extreme (1). According to Porritt (408), doping is an evil—it is morally wrong, physically dangerous, socially degenerate, legally indefensible, and an expression of an inferiority complex. Pawlucki (398) contends it is becoming a social disaster. In a more subdued opinion, Burt (79) indicated that the use of any drug in the athletic arena, for a nonmedical reason, is a refusal to live within one's natural limits, and usually represents a refusal to be individually responsible for one's own success or failure. Prokop (412), reporting for the International Federation of Sports Medicine (FISM) conference on doping, reiterated these general ethical and moral viewpoints.

Although Kourounakis (309) and Ariens (24) contend that pharmacological knowledge can be successfully applied to athletics, the paradox stems from the fact that most other sports medicine authorities (101, 134, 177, 228, 376, 387, 412) have concluded no pharmacological preparation can enhance human athletic performance. Prokop (412) stated his research with placebo tests presents possibly the most convincing evidence against doping. His research has indicated that the performance of top athletes was significantly improved following the intake of entirely inert substances provided the athlete believed them to be effective drugs. On the other hand, the administration of a potent compound provided no effect when they were designated as placebos. His experimentation demonstrates the effect of the power of suggestion and the essential ineffectiveness of drugs in athletics. Yet, in the same report, guidelines were established for banning certain drugs from athletics.

Thus, we have on one hand a concerted effort by most athletic governing bodies to legislate against the use of drugs in sports, and on the other hand, sports scientists propounding the relative ineffectiveness of drugs to increase performance. It would appear logical to the athlete to assume that if a certain drug is banned by the NCAA, IAAF, AAU or IOC, then it must be effective in enhancing performance. The sport ethic rationale seems to perpetuate this assumption. However, as Hoyman (260) indicated, we are in the midst of an ethical revolution, and the concept of situation ethics—the new morality—may be applicable to the doping problem. Some athletes are confronted with the antagonism between the winning is the only thing concept and the ethical issue of doping, and thus may consider the ethics of doping irrelevant in relation to winning.

In reality, if what sports scientists say is true regarding the ineffectiveness of doping, then there is no ethical issue. The main rationale against drug use in athletics is, therefore, health related, and this information should be stressed in the education of the athlete.

Theoretical Values of Drug Use in Athletics

If one attempted to evaluate the factors which are involved in athletic success, he would, after a few minutes deliberation, realize that sport is an extremely diverse field, and that the abilities characteristic of success in a particular sport or athletic activity may be extremely divergent. Considering just one aspect, body height, it is apparent that the taller man has an advantage in such activities as basketball, high jumping and putting the shot, but may be at a disadvantage in other sports such as gymnastics, since the strength to mass ratio is greater for a smaller man and consequently beneficial when lifting one's body weight.

There are numerous factors which contribute to success in a given event. Coaches and trainers use the terms aerobic capacity, strength, power, endurance, agility, hand-eye coordination, perceptual ability, motor ability, technique, motivation, anaerobic processes, tactics, intelligence, flexibility, dedication, concentration, and others of a physiological and psychological nature to describe those characteristics which an athlete must possess in order to be successful. It is obvious that all athletes do not possess these characteristics to the same degree, and that certain components are more prominent in one sport than another. For example, it is evident that the demands placed upon a professional golfer are extremely different from those necessary for success in running the mile; even in an activity as basic as running, the sprinter exhibits different physiological, and possibly psychological, characteristics than does the long-distance runner.

Thus, when one attempts to ascertain how drugs may affect performance in a given sport, he must identify what factors are involved in that sport and how drugs might beneficially modify them in order to increase athletic capacity. Sollman (486) has succinctly described the function of pharmacological agents by noting they rarely if ever create new functions in a cell or tissue, but simply modify existing functions or activate latent functions.

Several authors have constructed various classifications of sports based upon physiological and psychological characteristics, and the typology proposed by Vanek and Cratty (517) appears to be representative of the general demands placed upon athletes. The following classification is not restrictive, for an individual may need more than one of the general characteristics to be successful. Moreover, an individual participating in a sport such as football, with its many diversified positions, may be placed under a category dependent upon his position; the demands placed on the quarterback are much different than those on a tackle. The following discussion represents the typology of Vanek and Cratty with an integration of how drugs may hypothetically affect performance in the various categories.

1. *Sports involving hand-foot-eye coordination.* Activities such as golf, archery, riflery, place kicking in football, free throw shooting and tennis all require a definite muscular adjustment to visual clues. This adjustment may be subject to emotional stress of competition. Vanek and Cratty have indicated that athletes participating in such activities may use some type of depressant or tranquilizing drug prior to or during competition

in order to reduce the associated tension. Thus, psychodepressants may be beneficial if the mental condition of the athlete, such as anxiety, nervousness, or insomnia, is not under normal control.

2. *Sports involving total body coordination in a closed type activity.* Gymnastics and figure ice skating are examples of sports whereby the athlete performs alone without the interaction of others. Mixtures of amphetamines and barbiturates have been hypothesized to increase total body awareness while concomitantly decreasing tension.

3. *Sports involving use of body energy stores.* In aerobic activity, oxygen is the key to releasing body energy, and drugs such as cardiac stimulants, vasodilators, or oxygen carriers, which may increase maximal oxygen consumption, have been utilized. In addition, drugs which delay the subjective sensations of fatigue or counteract the accumulation of fatigue products have been proposed as ergogenic. The stimulants, aspartates, and alkalies might fall into this category.

4. *Sports involving the possibility of injury or death.* In motor car racing, alpine skiing and boxing, drugs which would have the purported effect of facilitating reaction time and movement time, or of making the individual more aware of the rapidly changing environment during the event, hypothetically could enhance performance. This effect has been attributed to amphetamines and other stimulants by several investigators.

5. *Sports which involve other individuals and perception of their possible movements.* Tennis, baseball and most team sports are categorized as open activities. A tremendous variety exists, and drugs which have been mentioned in the first four classifications, hypothetically, could be used in most team sports.

6. *Sports which are dependent upon muscle mass.* Although this is not a classification utilized by Vanek and Cratty, it is included because of the increased emphasis on strength in athletics. The relationship between muscle size and power has prompted weight lifters, shot putters and football players to maximize body development through the use of anabolic steroids. With the increasing importance of women's athletics, anabolic and androgenic steroids have been hypothesized to be of value,

even more so than in men's athletics. In addition, according to Klafs and Lyon (298), the female athlete has found that the menstrual cycle adversely affects her performance capacity. Thus, the use of the estrogen-progesterone oral contraceptives may be utilized to regulate the onset of her period.

Ultimate physical performance is the interaction of both physiological and psychological processes. All sports physiologists and psychologists agree that physiological factors set the relatively fixed and distal limits of performance, while psychological factors the more proximate ones. Bob Beaman had the physiological capacity for a 29+ foot long jump, and Jim Ryan could produce sufficient energy for a 3:51 mile—but how often do they perform at these levels? How often can athletes psych themselves for extreme effort? The ability to become highly self-motivated for competition—to psych oneself up—is an example of psychological processes inducing favorable physiological changes through increased secretion of adrenaline and sympathin. It is the natural way to stimulate the body to activity. Although Vanek and Cratty contend that superior athletes generally have a high degree of self control, and resist any technique which could tend to belittle their successful performance, it has nevertheless been reported that certain top athletes do resort to drugs in an attempt to reach physiological or psychological levels necessary for high caliber competition.

Craig (117) contends there is a finite limit to performance in athletic events which are measured in distance or time. Ultimate records will be approached asymptotically, with smaller and smaller increments, until the ultimate is reached. Since that zenith will always be there in man's mind, the athlete who believes he has done everything humanly possible to prepare for an event, may resort to some exogenous agent in an attempt to insure maximal effort. That exogenous agent may be a drug.

The following four chapters will present the available research relevant to the effectiveness of the variety of pharmacological agents which have been utilized in an attempt to increase the physical performance capacity of athletes.

CHAPTER 2

DRUGS AFFECTING THE NERVOUS SYSTEM—STIMULANTS

T HE BASIC PURPOSE of the nervous system is communication. Through the neural interrelationships between the sensorimotor aspects of both the CNS and the peripheral nervous system, each body cell is, theoretically, potentially able to communicate with every other body cell. Consequently, any drug affecting the CNS may exert widespread physiological and psychological responses. These responses might include stimulation or depression of muscular, respiratory or cardiovascular functions as well as the subjective state of the mind, and thus might influence human athletic performance.

A number of classifications have been developed to categorize CNS drugs dependent upon their physiological and/or psychological actions. Terms such as analgesic, hypnotic, sedative, tranquilizer, psychomotor, anti-depressant, psychotogenic, sympathomimetic, narcotic, hallucinogenic, and others are used to describe the basic pharmacological actions of certain drugs. However, most CNS drugs generally may be classified as either stimulants or depressants and are ranged on a continuum of potency. For example, both aspirin and morphine may be classified as depressants, yet one is extremely more potent than the other; the same is true of mild anti-depressants and strychnine in the stimulant category.

Stimulants and depressants mediate their effects by their actions on synapses throughout the various subdivisions of the

CNS. The transmission of an impulse across the synaptic gap involves the secretion of a neurohormone from the pre-synaptic fiber, diffusion across the gap, and a chemical reaction with the receptor cells on the post-synaptic fiber. Thus drugs may inhibit or accelerate production of the neurohormone, modify the rate of its dissolution or accumulation in the synaptic gap, or affect the post-synaptic receptors so the normal effect of the neurohormone is changed. Although the specific physiological and psychological effects of most common CNS drugs are fairly well known, the exact biochemical reactions and locus of action for many drugs remain to be completely resolved. While neurophysiologists are gradually unraveling the complexities of the nervous system, much is still unknown.

Drugs may mediate their effect on the CNS, and upon subsequent performance, in a variety of ways. If the cerebral cortex is affected, sensory perception, thinking, attention, motivation, motor responses and other cerebral activity may be changed dependent upon the area of the cortex involved. Sensory impulses to the cortex may be modified if the drug affects the ascending reticular activating system (ARAS), including the thalamus. The hypothalamus is concerned with control of the autonomic nervous system; it also influences the endocrine system via its relationship to the pituitary gland. In addition, the function of the hypothalamus is interrelated with the activity of the ARAS and such behavioral functions as wakefulness, alertness, excitability, pleasure, pain and rage. Thus, drugs affecting its function may produce widespread results. The medulla oblongata contains numerous clusters of cells, such as the vasomotor, cardiac and respiratory centers which may be influenced by drugs, while other drugs may exert their effect upon the spinal cord.

The most abused drugs in athletics are the CNS drugs, primarily those that exert a stimulating effect. However, depressants of various types have been utilized in conjunction with sports. In 1972, the Medical Commission of the International Olympic Committee proscribed the use of the following general classes of CNS drugs in conjunction with sports: CNS stimulants, sympathomimetic amines, the "caines" (cocaine, etc.), antidepressant agents, tranquilizers, pain pills, and narcotics such as morphine. As can be seen, both stimulants and depressants are included in the proscribed list. This chapter will include a discussion of the principal stimulants which have been utilized as an attempt to increase human performance capability.

In general, stimulants increase the excitability of the nerve cells in the CNS, facilitating the processes of both sensory input and motor output. Since the following drugs have been purported to increase work capacity or athletic performance by either a direct action on the CNS or through their sympathomimetic activity, they have been banned from use in athletic events by several athletic governing bodies:

amiphenazole	methylphenidate
amphetamine	methoxyphenamine
bemegride	methylephedrine
benzphetamine	nikethamide
cocaine	norpseudo ephedrine
diethylpropion	pemoline
dimethylamphetamine	phendimetrazine
ephedrine	phenmetrazine
ethylamphetamine	phentermine
fencamfamin	pipradol
fenproporex	prolintane
leptazole	strychnine
methylamphetamine	

In addition, any related compounds are also proscribed.

For purposes of discussion, the stimulants will be grouped into five classes: (a) amphetamines and similar agents, (b) cocaine, (c) caffeine and the xanthines, (d) nicotine, and (e) psychotomimetics.

AMPHETAMINES AND SIMILAR AGENTS

Probably the most abused class of drugs in athletics is amphetamines and related agents. In the literature, these drugs are categorized by such terms as CNS stimulants, sympathomimetic agents, psychomotor or psychotropic stimulants, respiratory stimulants, cerebral stimulants or antidepressants. Although the pharmacological actions of these drugs are complex, an attempt will be made to simplify their functions in relationship to physical activity. The drugs may increase overall CNS excitability, affect primarily one aspect of the CNS, exert a sympathomimetic effect, or elicit combined CNS stimulation and sympathomimetic actions. Thus pipradrol hydrochloride is classified as a CNS stimulant and not a sympathomimetic amine, nikethamide primarily influences respiratory activity through its influence on the respiratory centers in the medulla, ephedrine is noted for its sympathomimetic action, while amphetamine has combined CNS stimulation and sympathomimetic activity.

Although the mode of action of these stimulant drugs may vary, the basic purpose is to influence the nervous system to produce subjective or objective mental and physical changes which may increase performance capacity. Stimulants of the CNS may act directly or indirectly, or may exert both (bimodal) effects. Amphetamine and some of its derivatives exert a direct effect, stimulating activity of the post-ganglionic sympathetic nerves. Other agents such as the hydrazene derivatives function indirectly by inhibiting monoamine oxidases (MAOI agents), thus allowing accumulation of noradrenaline and other catecholamines in brain tissue. The response, such as increased attention, respiratory stimulation, cardiac stimulation, or anoretic action depends on which part of the CNS is affected. When a sympathomimetic effect is produced, the response of a particular sympathetic effector organ may be dependent upon whether it contains alpha or beta receptors. Theoretically, norepinephrine affects only those effector cells that have the alpha receptor, whereas epinephrine affects both. In general, alpha stimulation results in vasoconstriction in the arterioles of the skin and splanchinic area, cardioacceleration and increased blood pressure. Beta stimulation causes vasodilation in the muscles, cardioacceleration and increased myocardial strength resulting in increased cardiac output, and bronchial relaxation.

Use in Athletics

While the actions of specific stimulant drugs may vary, they are utilized because they elicit several or all of the following physiological actions which may have implications for increased performance capacity:

1. Increased cardiac output as a result of cardioacceleration and increased myocardial force.

2. Increased respiratory function due to effect on respiratory centers in the medulla.

3. Increased metabolic rate and oxygen uptake.

4. Increased muscle and liver glycogenolysis.

5. Increased blood levels of glucose and FFA.

6. Increased smooth muscle tone (vasoconstriction) of peripheral blood vessels in the cutaneous and splanchnic circulation.

7. Decreased smooth muscle tone (vasodilation) to skeletal musculature and respiratory system.

8. Increased cerebral activity resulting in increased attention and wakefulness.

For the interested reader, an excellent survey of the history, chemistry, kinetics, pathology and effects of the psychomotor stimulants is presented by Van Rossum (516). Earlier reviews by Hahn (224) and Eckstein and Abboud (147) are also very informative.

Adrenalin

It is a well known fact that the sympathetic nervous system is involved in the physiological adjustment to exercise (32, 284), and that the secretions of the sympathetic branch of the autonomic nervous system (sympathin) and hormones of the adrenal medulla (epinephrine and norepinephrine) are biochemically and metabolically similar. Consequently, some early research was conducted with the naturally occurring sympathomimetic amine, epinephrine, and its effect upon performance. Using trained dogs on a treadmill, Campos and his associates (83) revealed that although the injection of Adrenalin® before the start of exercise in rested animals raised the blood sugar level, it had no effect on the amount of work done by dogs. However, when Adrenalin was injected into the fatigued animals, they seemed to improve on a subsequent work task. This report may be analogous to more recent evidence that Adrenalin has no effect upon the isometric tension of the nonfatigued soleus muscle of the cat, but does increase the tension in the fatigued muscle (283). Dill and others (138) remarked that dogs evidently do not need extra supplies of Adrenalin in order to increase performance.

In more recent research, the infusion of epinephrine and norepinephrine into the heart of exercising dogs did not influence cardiac output, although the stroke volume increased with a concomitant decrease in heart rate; this finding may be indicative of increased cardiac efficiency (295). Marshall (346) studied the effect of infused epinephrine upon some cardiovascular and metabolic responses to leg exercise in man. Using a supine submaximal exercise test on a bicycle ergometer, epinephrine substantially increased blood flow to the legs as compared to exercise without epinephrine. However, the arteriovenous oxygen difference decreased during the epinephrine test, indicating that although the blood supply, and therefore the oxygen supply, to the muscle was increased, the muscles did not utilize the extra oxygen. This may be due to the fact that the exercise was submaximal; a different effect might occur during maximal exercise. Although no definite conclusion may be made relative to the effect of Adrenalin upon athletic performance, these few studies offer an indication that natural sympathomimetic amines may influence work output. However, in order for Adrenalin to be effective, it must be injected as it is hydrolyzed and rendered inactive if taken orally. If one believes that Adrenalin could facilitate athletic performance, then it would be useful to have it, or a similar compound, available in a capsule form for oral use. Hence, amphetamines and their congeners have become very popular in athletics.

Stimulants and Physical Working Capacity

Probably the most widely used, as well as controversial, drugs used in conjunction with athletics are the amphetamines and similar stimulants. A 1958 survey by the American College of Sports Medicine noted amphetamine was the most frequently mentioned drug in connection with sports (415), while Venerando

(518) implicated it on the European athletic scene. Gilbert (202, 203, 204) presented more recent evidence as to its predominance as the number one doping agent. Although amphetamine appears to be used extensively in sports, there are differing opinions regarding its use or effectiveness to increase performance capacity. Wallace (530) contended that as long as dosages are carefully controlled and under a doctor's prescription, small amounts are probably not dangerous and may actually be of help. Weiss and Laties (534) also indicated amphetamines are benign agents and their use may enhance performance. Other reports (16, 369) indicated amphetamines do improve performance. Based on these thoughts, most athletic governing bodies proscribe the use of amphetamines. As early as 1939, Boje (56) suggested they be banned from athletics, even though he indicated no investigations had been conducted relative to their effect upon muscular performance. In the past decade they have been condemned by the NCAA, AAU, IAAF, IOC as well as several major medical associations involved in the conduct of athletics. On the other hand, Segers and his colleagues (456) contended that amphetamine usage causes such a series of unfavorable physiological influences during exercise that its use in athletic performance is not only useless, but may be damaging as well. The Medical Commission of the 1970 British Commonwealth Games also noted amphetamines have not produced beneficial physiological changes during performance (354). Probably the soundest statement regarding amphetamines and athletics was propounded by Lovingood (332). He noted the basic question of whether amphetamine improves or fails to improve general physical performance has not been conclusively answered. The following review of experimental studies supports Lovingood's viewpoint.

Experimentation with Animals

Although the effects of drugs upon exercising animals cannot be extrapolated to man with complete validity, there are certain advantages associated with animal experimentation. Elimination of legal problems, more adequate control of extraneous variables which may interfere in human experimentation, condensed life span, similar genetic and environmental backgrounds, and the ability to sacrifice the animal for more detailed examination are but a few of the advantages. Aside from the extrapolation problem, the inability to communicate with the animal presents another disadvantage in contrast to human experiments. The primary animals used for research purposes concerning drugs and exercise performance have been rats and mice, although other species have been used. The basic performance test is usually swimming or running for speed or until exhaustion.

Swimming Tests. Amphetamine disrupted the starting performance in rats who were trained to start on a particular stimulus and swim an underwater tube to escape. Uyeno (515) hypothesized the delay was an indication of disrupted perception of the starting stimulus. Delayed perception would result in a slower speed. Kay and Birren (293) noted an improvement in the swimming speed of rates following Benzedrine, but indicated their results were inconclusive and further research was needed. Kleinrok and Swiezynska (301) found that 5 mg/kg amphetamine increased swimming speed in rats both with and without weights attached to their tails. On the other hand, Battig (42) noted 1.5 and 4 mg/kg dosages of amphetamine had no effect on the swimming velocity of unloaded rats, but produced a significant decrement in the weighted group. In an extensive study, Latz and his associates (317) investigated the effect of variant dosages (1, 2, 4 and 8 mg/kg) of d-amphetamine and other stimulants on swimming speed. The results indicated that relative to their own pre-treatment baselines, all treatments impaired swimming times. Swimming times were also slower after the placebo condition. However, relative to the placebo, the lower dosages of d-amphetamine and phenelzine facilitated speed. Latz contended that the placebo results suggest the drugs were tested on moderately fatigued animals, and that the most important aspect of interpretation of the drug effects is not with respect to the pre-treatment performance, but rather the placebo performance as compared to the post-treatment sessions. In reference to d-amphetamine, the smaller doses facilitated performance, but the larger dose (8 mg/kg) impaired the swimming time relative to placebo. The authors suggested that the main effect of d-amphetamine is on the energizing system, the lower dosages diminishing the effects of fatigue while the higher dosages augment the effects. Although a well-designed study, the interpretation that the drugs beneficially affect performance is predicated on the use of the placebo times, in contrast to the pre-treatment times, as the basis for evaluation. There may be a question as to whether or not this is a valid means to interpret the results of the experiment.

In summary, these studies indicate amphetamine may facilitate, impair, or have no effect upon swimming speed in animals.

Swim tests to exhaustion represent tests of endurance. Forcing mice to swim literally to death, Foldi-Borcsok and his associates (171) found that an unspecified stimulant, esberitox, increased their swimming endurance. The stimulant group had a mortality rate of 18 percent, compared to 37 percent for a saline group and 46 percent for the controls. Battig (42) noted that 4 mg/kg amphetamine increased the swimming endurance capacity of rats, while 1.5 mg/kg had no effect. In a previous report (41) and a summarization report of his animal studies (43), Battig stated amphetamines had no influence on tests of all-out physical effort. Jacob and Michaud (269) also noted amphetamine exerted no effect upon swim to exhaustion times in water at 20° C. In more recent research, Cooter (111) conducted a rather intricate study, testing the effect of 4, 8, 12 and 16 mg/kg of dl-amphetamine sulfate, administered 30, 60, 90 or 120 minutes prior to testing, upon the endurance swimming performance of twenty-three rats. A control situation was also used. All rats underwent all seventeen conditions. The ANOVA revealed no significant differences between the experimental treatments and control; hence, Cooter concluded swimming endurance was not enhanced by amphetamines. In a similar study, Rokosz (433) evaluated the effect of 5 and 10 mg/kg of d-amphetamine sulfate on rats swimming to exhaustion; tests were conducted following three time periods (20, 40 and 60 minutes). A control trial was also included in the design; thus, each rat was exposed to seven tests. The results indicated that d-amphetamine sulfate produced a 50 percent decrement in performance. However, there was no significant difference between the two dosages or time levels.

In general, the results of these studies support the concept that amphetamine does not significantly influence swimming endurance capacity of animals.

Running Tests. Daily oral doses of 10 mg/kg of 2-ethylamino-3-phenyl-norcamphane-hydrochloride (H610) reportedly increased the muscular performance in rats who were forced to run to exhaustion on a rotating drum. Sommer and Hotovy (487) suggested that improved economy of muscular coordination as the result of central stimulation was an important determining factor in the increased performance levels. Studying the effect of various dosages (0.3, 1.0, 2.0, 3.0, and 5.0 mg/kg) of methylamphetamine on blood lactate levels in rats after a standardized prolonged exercise task, Chaterjee and his associates (91) reported a U effect, i.e. low and high dosages eliciting high blood lactic acid levels whereas moderate doses depressed them. They concluded that optimal doses of methylamphetamine improved physical work efficiency by preventing a rise in blood lactic levels after exercise. It appears in this study that individual t-tests were used to compare differences between groups, when a one-way ANOVA and multiple range test may have been more appropriate and may have changed the interpretation of the data. Although Stewart (492) reported a tendency towards increased speed in racehorses receiving 0.2 mg/kg amphetamine, his results were not statistically significant.

In summary, the results regarding the effect of stimulants upon the running performance of animals are equivocal, due both to the paucity of research and the nature of the studies reviewed above.

Experimentation with Humans

Numerous studies have been conducted regarding the effect of amphetamines upon human performance. Those reviewed have been categorized into subjective effects, effects upon psychomotor performance, effects upon physiological modifications during exercise, influence upon strength and local muscular endurance, effect on general endurance, and effects upon field tests of athletic skills.

Subjective Effects. In general, amphetamines produce a subjective psychological state of excitability, which has been postulated as the rationale for improved performance in athletics. Cameron and associates (82), through an extensive longitudinal questionnaire analysis, reported the general effects of amphetamines on moods, emotions and motivation caused their subjects to be more energetic. Testing other stimulants in addition to amphetamine, Martin (347) used a double-blind placebo design and reported the separate use of d-amphetamine, d-methamphetamine, phenmetrazine, methylphenidate, and ephedrine elicited a general euphorogenic response with feelings of general excitability and increased confidence. Shah and associates (460) found similar effects of d-amphetamine sulfate and norcamphane hydrochloride in reducing the subjective symptoms of fatigue associated with repetitious work. In a study dealing specifically with athletes, Smith and Beecher (480) used the questionnaire method to investigate the effect of amphetamine upon the athlete's subjective evaluation of his performance, mood state and physical state. They reported the athletes could distinguish the amphetamines from placebos and secobarbital, and in general expressed sensations of increased mental and physical stimulation. The peak subjective and behavioral effects were evidenced 2 to 3 hours after the ingestion of approximately 14 mg amphetamine. However, in a follow-up report (481), most athletes did not feel they went all out on amphetamine days as contrasted to placebo days. Thus, no positive conclusion was made relative to the effect of amphetamine upon the athlete's judgment of his performance.

Summarizing from his own research in this field, Battig (43) concluded it is unjustifiable to view amphetamines as a direct stimulant of performance. Rather, his studies indicate amphetamine is only a psychotropic drug, which, by its action on the higher CNS functions may lift the subjective limits of performance, and thus possibly remove normal inhibitions which may restrict athletic capacity.

Effect Upon Psychomotor Performance. A number and variety of psychological and psychomotor tests are available. Speed of tapping, object manipulation, hand steadiness, balance, tracking, visual perception, speed of vision, attentive ability, and other such tests have been utilized in order to evaluate the effects of drugs upon perceptual-motor ability (156, 169, 241, 251, 252, 300, 333, 406, 414, 497, 506). Of the variety of psychomotor tests available, the most used, and probably the one most applicable to athletics, involves the measurement of reaction time and/or movement time.

Using sleep-deprived or fatigued subjects, several investigators (307, 454, 511) reported beneficial effects of amphetamines upon reaction time, while Cuthbertson and Knox (124) noted no difference. In an older study with rested subjects, Thornton and his colleagues (506) evaluated the effect of 20 mg amphetamine upon performance in nine psychomotor tests. The results indicated amphetamine produced a faster reaction time. Although the experimental design was quite good, the interpretation of the data with only three subjects may have produced an erroneous conclusion. Using a more controlled double-blind placebo design, with more sophisticated recording equipment and more subjects, Rasch and others (415) concluded that 20 mg amphetamine, a commonly used dosage associated with competitive athletics, had no effect on human reaction time or movement time in response to a visual stimulus. In support of Rasch and his colleagues, Kornetsky (306) reported that neither 5 nor 15 mg d-amphetamine had any significant effect upon simple or choice reaction time. Lovingood and his associates (333) also reported that 5 mg amphetamine had no effect on visual reaction time. However, in a later study, Lovingood (331) reported a significantly faster simple reaction time following ingestion of 15 mg amphetamine. The difference in dosages may have been the deciding factor.

Wenzel and Rutledge (538) reported evidence contrary to that of Rasch and his colleagues. They evaluated the effect of several stimulants upon both simple visual and complex reaction time; drugs and dosages included d-amphetamine (2.5, 5.0 and

10.0 mg), phenmetrazine (12.5, 25.0 and 50.0 mg), and methyl phenidyl acetate (5, 10, and 15 mg). The general conclusion indicated all stimulants produced improvements in both tests. The design of this study was quite complex, as was their discussion of the results, which appeared to contradict the general conclusion noted above.

The literature regarding the effect of amphetamine upon reaction time appears to be contradictory. Consequently, more specific research is needed in this area since reaction time has been associated with success in athletics (268).

Effect on Physiological Adjustments to Exercise. In a resting state the ingestion of amphetamine has been shown to increase the heart rate, respiratory rate, oxygen uptake, blood lactate levels, and blood pressure (259, 347, 456). During exercise the sympathetic nervous system elicits similar effects; thus, a variety of studies have been conducted to determine whether amphetamine has an augmenting effect on cardiovascular, respiratory and metabolic adjustments to exercise.

Concerning the heart rate response to submaximal exercise, several investigators (402, 548) reported no significant change in contrast to control trials, whereas others reported significant increases (37, 38, 261, 331, 333, 386, 456, 469, 476, 519). The findings relative to maximal heart rate are also contradictory as Margaria and his associates (341) reported no significant effect of amphetamine (10 mg) during a maximal treadmill test, while Williams and Thompson (548) reported a significant increase during a maximal bicycle ergometer test following the ingestion of three different dosages (5, 10 and 15 mg/70 kg). However, they did indicate this finding could be a chance occurrence.

The increased heart rate, provided stroke volume remained constant, would be indicative of an increased cardiac output. Only one study was uncovered which evaluated the effect of a stimulant upon exercise cardiac output. Silverman and his colleagues (469) noted a significant increase in cardiac output under the influence of isoprenaline; the change was due to heart rate increases as the stroke volume remained unchanged; also, there was no indication whether the workload was maximal or submaximal.

Probably one of the best single physiological indicators of physical working capacity is maximal oxygen consumption. If this parameter could be increased through amphetamine ingestion, it might be indicative of greater aerobic power and the ability to produce more aerobic energy during work. On the other hand, increased levels of oxygen uptake at standardized submaximal work would represent decreased mechanical efficiency. One report (456) noted a significant increase in submaximal oxygen uptake due to amphetamine, while Osness (386) indicated a slight increase during submaximal work and the greatest increase during maximal work; however, levels of significance were not given in the brief abstract available. The majority of reports signify no significant influences of amphetamine upon submaximal or maximal oxygen consumption. Bartak and Skranc (38), Pirnay and his colleagues (402), and Venerando (520) found no effect on submaximal oxygen uptake, while Margaria and others (341) reported no influence on maximal oxygen uptake.

Minute ventilation (37, 38, 469), respiratory rate (38, 386), ventilatory equivalent (523), oxygen pulse (524), respiratory quotient (522), and CO_2 production (37, 386, 521) were not significantly affected by amphetamine or similar agents during exercise. Osness (386), however, did report slight increases in minute ventilation.

Increased levels of blood lactic acid following exercise would suggest the subject is deriving more energy from anaerobic sources. If the increased level occurred during submaximal exercise, one might hypothesize the individual is inefficient, since anaerobic work is less efficient than aerobic work. If greater blood lactate levels are found at maximal exercise, the same conclusion may be made provided the maximal work loads were identical. However, if the subject can sustain a higher maximal work load, he may possibly do so because of increased ability to utilize anaerobic sources of energy, i.e. glycolysis which will increase blood lactate. Bartak and Skranc reported no significant influence of stimulants on blood lactate levels following heavy (38) or maximal (37) work; two stimulants, 50 mg dexfenmetrazin and 20 mg psychoton were utilized in both experiments. On the other hand, Pirnay and others (402) reported a significant effect of amphetamine (25 mg) on blood lactate levels three hours after a maximal exercise test. The authors indicated this may be proof of an augmented anaerobic metabolism and may be a factor involved in the improvement of performance. However, a complicating factor, which may affect their interpretation, is the fact that no significant differences in blood lactate levels were noted thirty minutes following the termination of the exercise test. In a study involving the effect of 10 mg amphetamine upon endurance capacity of two highly trained bicyclists, Wyndham and others (554) reported a significant increase in blood lactic acid during maximal exercise as a result of amphetamine ingestion. Both subjects did more work under the influence of amphetamine, and the authors attributed this effect to increased anaerobic capacity. However, blood lactate levels were only obtained for one subject; thus, there is only a population of one from which the general conclusion has been made. With six subjects, Hueting and Poulus (261) noted amphetamines appeared to increase blood lactate levels following maximal work. It is unlikely that amphetamine directly improves anaerobic capacity, but possibly through its effect to delay fatigue sensations, the subjects were able to continue work longer and accumulate more lactic acid.

In summary, with the possible exception of the heart rate response to submaximal exercise, and blood lactate levels following maximal exercise, the majority of other physiological adjustments to exercise do not appear to be significantly influenced by amphetamine. Even if amphetamine elicited a hypothetically favorable cardiovascular, respiratory, or metabolic response during exercise, it would not only be difficult, but imprudent, to extrapolate this to the athletic arena unless the event in question was dependent primarily upon the particular physiological parameter involved. Thus far, no favorable modification of physiological parameters associated with exercise has been definitely substantiated for amphetamine and similar stimulants.

Effect Upon Strength and Local Muscular Endurance. Muscular strength and endurance are important factors in most athletic events. It is obvious, therefore, that drugs to improve these parameters might be employed by athletes. Lovingood and his colleagues (333) reported that 5 mg d-amphetamine, in contrast to a placebo, had no significant effect on total body strength as represented by the summation of isometric handgrip, back and leg lifts on a dynamometer. In a later double-blind placebo study, Lovingood (331) employed a larger dose (15 mg d-amphetamine) and found a significant increase in left hand grip strength. Graham and Bos (216) also reported a significant increase in isometric strength following the ingestion of 15 mg amphetamine. Studying the effect of various factors modifying the expression of human strength, Ikai and Steinhaus (264) reported a statistically significant improvement in isometric forearm strength twenty-five minutes following the ingestion of 30 mg amphetamine. Danysz (127) also reported increased dynamometer strength levels after amphetamine. In comparison with a placebo, Adamson and Finley (4) indicated a newly developed stimulant, WIN·19,583 (200 mg) and amphetamine (10 mg) both effectively increased static strength as measured on spring steel and hydraulic dynamometers. They also noted the new stimulant appeared to be more effective than amphetamine. In summary, the results of these studies suggest amphetamines increase isometric strength. No evidence was uncovered regarding the effect of amphetamine upon isotonic, or dynamic, strength.

The effect of amphetamine upon muscular endurance is debatable. Using a Mosso-type finger ergograph, Alles and Feigen (14) investigated the effect of 10, 20, and 40 mg amphetamine upon local muscular endurance. They concluded amphetamine inhibits the production of voluntary fatigue, as indicated by an increase in the extent and number of muscular contractions on the ergograph recording. However, the number of subjects was small (N=6) and no counterbalancing of order of drug administration was done; the control trial was done first in all cases. Thus, a biased motivational device may have been in operation, i.e. to outperform one's previous trial. Other complicating factors render the interpretation of their data questionable. Bujas and Petz (74) measured the effect of 15 mg amphetamine on the ability of eighteen subjects to maintain an 8.5 kg load in a test of static endurance. The results indicated amphetamine increased isometric endurance as compared to placebo. Similar results were obtained by Graham and Bos (216). In a well-designed double-blind placebo experiment, they studied the effect of 15 mg d-amphetamine upon isometric and isotonic muscular endurance of the triceps brachii; muscle action potentials were recorded concurrently. They found that d-amphetamine significantly decreased the integrated action potentials and local fatigue of the triceps during isometric contractions, but had no significant effect during the isotonic contractions. Graham and Bos concluded that, with certain limitations, d-amphetamine will not significantly delay the onset of muscular fatigue in most cases of muscular work during athletics, as the majority of sports involves isotonic, and not isometric, work. Adamson and Finley (4) substantiate this viewpoint as they found no significant effect of 10 mg amphetamine or 200 mg WIN·19,583 upon isotonic endurance; maximal execution of pull-ups was the criterion measure of muscular endurance.

Costello (113) investigated the effect of 10 mg d-amphetamine on the ability to sustain two-thirds maximal strength level as long as possible on a hand dynamometer. Using five conditions (amphetamine, two tranquilizers, placebo and control), a significant F ratio was obtained for the drug effect. Follow up statistical tests revealed the only significant difference was between the control and d-amphetamine. These results indicate amphetamine does not affect endurance, and substantiates the importance for inclusion of a placebo treatment in drug experimentation. Using women as subjects in the same experimental design, Costello indicated amphetamine elicited higher muscular endurance values when compared to the other four conditions. Using a hand dynamometer, Singh (475) reported no significant difference between placebo and d-amphetamine on muscular endurance. He did note, however, that the mean values for amphetamine were lower than the placebo condition. Using an arm hang test as a criterion of muscular endurance, Bujas and others (75) reported no significant influence of several different stimulants.

Effect on General Endurance. While the preceding section dealt partly with local muscular endurance, the following discussion centers on general endurance of large muscular groups, primarily involving tests of cardiovascular-respiratory endurance although local muscular endurance is important in both bicycle ergometer and incline treadmill work. In one of the earliest studies evaluating the effect of amphetamine upon general endurance, Lehman and his associates (322) noted that amphetamine enabled greater work ability in tests to exhaustion on a bicycle ergometer. Knoefel (303) used a progressive work load on the bicycle ergometer as his criterion test. Both amphetamine and Pervitin® (desoxyephedrine) were used, with dosages of 10 and 20 mg, along with a placebo trial. Although no statistical analysis was presented, one subject had a 60 percent increase in work capacity with the stimulants, four others had smaller increases, and two were unaffected by the dosages. In a more recent study, Wyndham and others (554) also reported a 61 percent increase in maximal work capacity of one subject following 10 mg methamphetamine; their second subject experienced a 29 per cent increase. However, run to exhaustion was based on a percentage of the subjects' max VO_2, and the authors do not indicate whether the absolute workload was the same under placebo and drug conditions. The increase was attributed to euphoria or increased threshold to pain, thus permitting the cyclists to derive more energy from anaerobic sources. Although it is hazardous to generalize from such a small population, the investigators did use highly trained bicyclists, a prerequisite when evaluating the effects of drugs upon athletic performance.

In other concurring reports, Osness (386) noted a slight increase in work capacity on a bicycle ergometer following 15 mg d-amphetamine, although he did not indicate whether the increase was significant or not. Bartak and Skranc (38) reported both dexfenmetrazin (50 mg) and psychoton (20 mg) significantly prolonged the work time of subjects exercising at 85 percent max VO_2. Cuthbertson and Knox (124) found that 15 mg amphetamine increased the capacity to sustain work on a bicycle ergometer. However, the workload was light (600 kgm), only six subjects were used and the authors noted wide individual variation; no statistical analysis was offered. Bujas and associates (75) indicated that stimulants such as Phenamine and Ritalin® had no positive effect on the treadmill or bicycle ergometer performance of subjects who were in a state of physical freshness and motivated for work; however, they did note there may be a certain positive effect of pharmacological stimulants in the final phase of maximal physical efforts. Borg and others (58) reported similar findings. They evaluated the effect of 10 mg amphetamine upon a series of intermittent and maximal work of short duration on a cycling strength and endurance test (CSET). The CSET was comprised of ten working periods of maximal performance, each lasting approximately forty-five seconds with a rest period of fifteen seconds between trials. Thirty-four subjects were pretested without drugs, and then assigned to one of three groups (amphetamine, amobarbital and placebo). The drugs were administered thirty, sixty, and thirty minutes, respectively, before the second CSET. The results indicated that amphetamine did not affect the initial performances in the second CSET, but improved performance towards the end of the test. Thus, amphetamines did not influence performance in a rested state, but may have been effective as fatigue set in.

Although the studies cited in the preceding paragraph support the contention that amphetamines improve general endurance capacity, possibly being more effective in the fatigued state, a number of contemporary experiments do not concur. Even in an older report, Foltz and others (174) found no influence of 10 mg amphetamine upon total bench stepping time to exhaustion in untrained subjects. Noting the confounding effects of training, the authors (175) conducted a subsequent study with trained subjects. Using a bicycle ergometer workload of 1235 kgm/minute, they investigated the effect of 10 to 15 mg amphetamine and 5 mg desoxyephedrine upon endurance in both a rested and fatigued condition; the subjects worked to exhaustion, rested ten minutes, and then worked to exhaustion again. Amphetamine did not affect performance in either work task, whereas desoxyephedrine increased output in the nonfatigued state, but not during the fatigued state. However, these two early reports had methodological deficiencies. In a run to exhaustion on a treadmill operating at a speed of 7.2 MPH and a 5 percent grade, Karpovich (288) reported that 10 mg amphetamine taken one hour prior to the test had no significant effect on endurance or recuperation performance of twenty-five subjects who took the test six times, three with placebo and three with amphetamine.

More recently, Margaria and others (341) found that 10 mg amphetamine did not increase the work capacity of three trained subjects; the criterion test was time to exhaustion on a treadmill at 12 to 13.8 km/hour with a 5 percent incline. The experiment was well designed as each subject was tested five times under drug and placebo conditions. In another sound study, Golding and Barnard (210) investigated the effect of 15 mg d-amphetamine on performance as measured by all-out treadmill running times at a speed of 10 MPH with a 8.5 percent grade. The drug was administered 2 to 3 hours prior to testing. The basic design consisted of two all-out runs on each test day; the second run, or fatigued run, was twelve minutes after the rested run. The subjects were ten track men and ten unconditioned college students. Tests were administered six times to the conditioned men (three drug and three placebo) and twice to the unconditioned subjects. The results showed that d-amphetamine sulfate exerted no significant effect on all-out runs performed in either a rested or fatigued state by conditioned or unconditioned subjects. Bartak and Skranc (37) reported no significant effect of 50 mg dexfenmetrazin or 20 mg psychoton, in contrast to placebo and no drug conditions, upon maximal work capacity on a bicycle ergometer; the mean maximal load was 345 watts. Hueting and Poulus (261) tested the effect of variant dosages of methylamphetamine (0, 10, 20, and 30 mg) upon the endurance capacity of six subjects; work consisted of a progressive bicycle ergometer test to exhaustion. The authors concluded amphetamine exerted no influence on performance when compared with placebo. In a similar study, Williams and Thompson (548) studied the actions of a placebo and three dosages (5, 10, and 15 mg/70 kg) of d-amphetamine upon a progressive bicycle ergometer ride to exhaustion. They concluded that variant dosages of d-amphetamine sulfate do not influence maximal endurance capacity.

In summary, the effects of stimulant drugs such as amphetamine upon the physical expression of strength and endurance is still unresolved. The drugs do appear to increase isometric strength, but evidence is contradictory relative to the influence upon local muscular and general endurance.

Effect Upon Athletic Performance—Field Tests. The amount of reported research concerning the direct effect of amphetamine upon actual competitive athletic performance is extremely limited, as are the number of studies which involve field testing. The answer is understandable. Aside from the legality problem involved with the use of drugs in actual competition, not too many coaches or others involved in the management of athletics would allow their athletes to use amphetamine because it has been classified as a dangerous drug. Moreover, an athlete who inadvertently might improve his field performance while involved in experimentation with the drug may believe it will enhance his performance in future events. There are probably other justifiable reasons, but if a conclusive answer relative to the effect of amphetamines upon human performance is to be revealed, athletes are necessary subjects.

Girdano and Girdano (205) contended that the popularity of amphetamine use in athletics is due to the lack of understanding or misunderstanding of research reports, and indicated that little research has been conducted on amphetamines and performance in the past ten years. They noted that simple repeatable measures such as swimming, running, and throwing might be improved by amphetamines, but that performance in complex skill activities such as basketball may deteriorate due to chemical hyperexcitability with reduction in coordination and concentration. The former supposition is probably extracted from the research of Smith and Beecher (479), a controversial report. No substantive evidence has been presented to support the latter statement regarding complex activities; this represents the extrapolation of amphetamine effects on simple psychomotor components, such as hand steadiness, to complex motor activities and is generally unwarranted.

Although not involved directly with athletics, two older studies revealed conflicting results on field performance. Sommerville (488) reported that 15 and 35 mg amphetamine did not enhance performance of fatigued soldiers on an obstacle course, whereas Seashore and Ivy (454) reported beneficial effects of Benzedrine on fatigued subjects undertaking a battery of physical performance tests.

In one of the earliest studies investigating the influence of amphetamine (5 mg) and another stimulant, Metrazol® (100 mg), upon athletic performance, Haldi and Wynn (226) reported no beneficial effect of these drugs upon the 100 yard swimming test for speed in twelve men. Although the mean time for the amphetamine condition was 0.6 seconds faster, the difference was not statistically significant. Karpovich (288) also studied the effect of amphetamine upon swimming performance. Using a dosage of 10 mg and criterion swim tests of 100, 220 and 440 yards, the amphetamine produced no significant alterations in eighteen swimmers. Using the same basic experimental design, Karpovich also reported no significant effect upon the competitive running performance (100 yards to two-mile runs) of eleven track men. On the other hand, Danysz and his coworkers (127) indicated a beneficial effect on performance in a 100 meter dash following the chronic administration of 2-dimethylaminethanol; dosages were 100 to 200 mg or 150 to 300 mg daily for two weeks.

Probably the most extensive, and most cited, report concerning the effects of amphetamine on the performance of athletes was conducted by Smith and Beecher, and presented in three separate reports in the *American Medical Association Journal* (479, 480, 481). They studied the influence of a 14 mg/70 kg dosage, administered 2 to 3 hours prior to testing, on the performance of highly trained swimmers, runners, and weight throwers. Their report actually consisted of six separate experiments, and included experimentation not only with amphetamine, but also secobarbital, a depressant. The secobarbital was used primarily to mask subjective effects of the amphetamines. The first experiment involved fifteen trained athletes who swam either a 100 or 200 yard event twelve times, four each with placebo, 14 mg amphetamine/70 kg, and 100 mg secobarbital. Experiments 2 to 4 involved experienced runners. Different subjects were in each group, and the distances covered ranged from 440 yards to 12.7 miles. These subjects ran a particular distance approximately three times under each condition, although the secobarbital dose was only 50 mg/70 kg. In the running experiment with the marathoners, additional dosages of 7 and 21 mg amphetamine were tested. The fifth experiment involved thirteen weight throwers and shot putters in their particular events. They took the same dosages as the runners. The sixth experiment involved sixteen swimmers, thirteen who participated in the first experiment. No secobarbital was used in this experiment; the amphetamine dose was 14 mg. All in all, eighteen swimmers were tested 453 times, twenty-six runners were tested 205 times, and the thirteen weight men performed 123 times.

The swimmers were the most extensively studied and the results showed a statistically significant increase in performance of short distance events (100 and 200 yards) following amphetamine ingestion. Smith and Beecher concluded that running performance is improved by amphetamines. Similar conclusions were made regarding the performances of the weight men in the field events. In general, Smith and Beecher concluded that amphetamine ingestion improved performance in diverse athletic events. In a subsequent study, Smith and others (482) reported similar results for nonexpert swimmers.

Although their study has been the most extensive field research project ever conducted relative to the effects of amphetamine upon athletic performance, it was not free from criticism. Pierson (400) indicated serious defects in the collection of the data, statistical techniques and interpretation of the results, while Shephard (466) also noted the results are still disputed. Among the many problems were different environmental conditions for the runners; the temperature ranged from 25° to 69° F and the wind velocity varied between 8 to 23 MPH. Some data was rejected due to strong winds or fatigue from a severe run the preceding day. The authors also indicated at one point there were reasons to question the validity of the data and yet they retained it. Other complicating factors included the utilization of an extrinsic motivational device and self-timing by some runners. Furthermore, rather unconventional levels of significance were used. The authors do comment on the methodological problems associated with their experimental design, and they also include relevant comments throughout the report. In spite of this, they concluded that the performance of highly trained athletes, of the classes studied, can be significantly improved in the majority of cases (about 75%) by the administration of amphetamine. However, they do contend that their findings do not prove that athletes competing in intercollegiate meets would be helped by amphetamines since they did not test under actual intercollegiate competition, although experiment six was conducted under similar competitive conditions.

The critical reader is referred to the excellent critique by Pierson (400) and the rejoinder by Cochran, Smith and Beecher (103). Moreover, he should digest the three part report and make his own interpretation.

Amphetamine and Temperature Regulation During Exercise

Disturbance of temperature regulation is one of the possible dangers associated with the use of amphetamines and other sympathomimetics during exercise. The deaths of several European bicyclists have been attributed to heat stroke, elicited through the synergistic action of amphetamines and high environmental temperature. In an experiment with mice, Hardinge and others (233) suggested that amphetamines interfere with temperature regulation. Animals forced to exercise died of a much lower dose of amphetamine than did unexercised animals; thus, hyperthermia and the associated mortality in amphetamine poisoning in mice appeared to be due to a combination of increased motor activity and impaired temperature regulation. Nikethamide, a potent respiratory stimulant, has been reported to exert a hyperthermia in the guinea pig, augmenting the hyperthermia induced by muscular effort. Frommel and his colleagues (187) indicated this may be due to the close interdependence of the respiratory, vasomotor and thermoregulatory centers. Lovingood and others (333) studied the effect of 5 mg d-amphetamine upon heat gain and sweat loss of human subjects during intermittent 1½ hours exercise in a three hour period; the exercise task consisted of treadmill walking at 4 MPH at 110° F. Amphetamine had no effect on either parameter. Shephard (466) noted that amphetamines could expose the athlete to a dangerous level of heat stress, since one of their actions is to constrict cutaneous arterioles; cutaneous vasodilation is necessary for heat elimination.

Based on the available evidence, it would appear prudent for the athlete who is illegally utilizing amphetamines to restrain from this practice during prolonged activity in environmental conditions that impose a heat stress.

As a side point, Zalis (557) indicated that although the lethal acute dose of amphetamine in the adult has been stated as 20 to 25 mg/kg, estimates from animal studies have suggested it may be as low as 5 mg/kg. In one case, a young man died from 140 mg methamphetamine.

Summarizing Statement

Probably the most accurate summarizing statement that can be made regarding the effect of amphetamines and related stimulants upon physical work capacity or athletic ability would involve guarded skepticism. As an illustration, two authorities recently reviewed the literature on this topic and came up with two entirely different opinions. Weiss (533) stated the evidence overwhelmingly favors the conclusion that amphetamine is able to enhance a wide variety of performances, ranging from simple psychomotor tasks to vigilance and physical endurance, especially in athletic events. On the contrary, Vidacek (528) evaluated both field and laboratory research and concluded that the effect of amphetamines and other sympathomimetics upon physical work output seems so negligible that it is easily masked by such other factors as individual subject differences and degree of motivation.

The solution to the dilemma is a concerted program of sound research. Two of the complicating factors in the evaluation of the literature involves dosage and elapsed time between ingestion and exericse. Several investigators indicated that there exists an optimal time and dose; however, neither has been completely substantiated.

Although the effects of stimulants upon athletic performance are controversial at the present time, there is one striking observation that should be made known. In the numerous studies that have been reviewed, amphetamine rarely caused a decrement in performance. Nevertheless, based upon this literature review, primarily the more contemporary laboratory research, it is concluded that amphetamines do not have any beneficial effect on athletic performance.

COCAINE

The stimulating effect of chewing coca leaves has been evident from the sixteenth century. The Spanish conquistadors discovered the Inca civilization in Peru used the coca leaves as their currency. Leaf chewing was a common practice, as the natives continuously had a wad of leaves in their mouths as they worked. Numerous reports have indicated the Indians could work for days, travel hundreds of miles, and withstand bitter cold without any sustenance except the coca leaves. The active ingredient was cocaine. Cuiffardi (121) reported the actual uptake of cocaine from the practice of chewing coca leaves was, on the average, 112 mg per quid, which is about 12 mg above the maximal recommended single dose. Habitual Indian chewers use several quids per day. The major portion must be absorbed through the oral mucosa, as the gastrointestinal tract inactivates cocaine. An extract from coca leaves was utilized in various commercial preparations throughout Europe during the nineteenth century, and was even used in America's favorite, Coca-Cola®, at the end of the nineteenth and beginning of the twentieth century (416). An early advertisement stated, in part, Coca-Cola . . . contains the valuable tonic and nerve stimulant properties of the coca plant and cola nuts (262). When the potential dependence hazards of cocaine were discovered, its use was eliminated from such compounds designed for everyday consumption. However, its effect in producing a sense of exhilaration was the main reason for the popularity of cocaine. In the brilliant biography of Freud, *The Passions of the Mind*, Stone (494) noted the psychoanalyst used it for a brief period of time because it increased his vitality and capacity for work.

Cocaine is an alkaloid derivative of the coca plant, erythroxylon coca. Therapeutically it is used extensively as a local anaesthetic, as it prevents transmission of impulses along nerve fibers and at nerve endings. Systemically, cocaine stimulates the cerebral cortex and gives rise to a feeling of well-being, with the sensation that the capacity for work is increased and fatigue may be postponed. Van Rossum (516) stated cocaine has a different mode of action than amphetamine, in that it potentiates the action of noradrenalin by inhibiting the re-uptake of noradrenalin in sympathetic neurons. Also in contrast to amphetamines, its duration of action is much shorter, the exhilarating effect lasting only 5 to 15 minutes. Consequently, repeated dosages must be consumed if a continued effect is desired; this may account for the constant coca chewing of the Andean Indians.

There is very little literature available relative to the use of cocaine in athletics. Boje (56) contended that cocaine, in conjunction with athletics, removes the sensation of fatigue and thus will undoubtedly raise the level of performance in events characterized by prolonged effort. This contention appears to be based upon his interpretation of experimentation by Mosso, who reported small doses of cocaine increased the capacity for muscular work on a finger ergograph. Theil and Essing (502), in 1933, also reported increased work capacity on a bicycle ergometer following the use of cocaine. However, the methodology of these early work experiments renders the interpretation of the data suspect. In more recent general statements, although without any elaboration on the source of information, Shephard (466) commented that cocaine may postpone fatigue and increase the endurance of cyclists, and Cohen (104) indicated occasional instances whereby cocaine had increased motor performance in athletes.

The available hard experimental data is limited. Jacob and Michaud (269) reported a stimulating dose of cocaine had no effect on the swim time to exhaustion in mice. Using Quechua Indians of Peru as subjects, Hanna (229) investigated the hypothesis that coca chewing enhances working ability. Six chewers and six nonchewers were used in his experiment. One hour prior to the work test, the coca chewers chewed coca in any desired quantity; the nonchewers had no treatment. Using four different standardized submaximal workloads on step benches, no significant differences were noted between the groups for ventilation and oxygen consumption, but the heart rates were lower and the blood pressure higher for the coca chewers. Hanna reported that the small number of subjects precluded firm conclusions, since the differences noted could have been due to sample variability. Using a better experimental design in a follow-up study, Hanna (230) recruited chewers and nonchewers, and had both groups take submaximal and maximal tests with and without coca. Thus, each subject served as his own control. Order of administration of the treatments was counterbalanced. Habitual chewers were given as much coca as they normally took, while the nonchewers were given 4 to 5 grams, the same amount normally used by chewers. The submaximal test consisted of a progressive consecutive twelve minute workload on a bicycle ergometer, three minutes each at 350, 525, 875, and 1150 kpm/minute; the maximal test began at 1050 kpm/minute for two minutes and was increased 175 kpm/minute until exhaustion. Parameters included oxygen consumption, ventilation, heart rate, systolic and diastolic blood pressures. During maximal work, time to exhaustion was an additional parameter. The results indicated that submaximal exercise heart rate was significantly higher when the subjects chewed coca; no other physiological parameters were significantly differentiated during submaximal or maximal work. During maximal work, although the duration of effort was not significantly increased, there was a mean difference of twenty seconds favoring the coca trial. Hanna indicated this is noteworthy, since it tends to support earlier empirical observations. He contended that cocaine potentiates the action of epinephrine and norepinephrine, which are normally increased during exercise, thus alleviating the sensation of fatigue. However, Hanna concluded that coca had no influence on work capacity.

From the limited evidence available, it would appear that cocaine has no effect on physical working capacity.

CAFFEINE

Caffeine is found in a variety of flora throughout the world; it is a CNS stimulant, affecting the cerebral cortex, medulla oblongata and spinal cord. Resultant subjective symptoms include increased wakefulness and mental activity (454). Caffeine may also stimulate the cardiac muscle, and increase respiratory rate and depth. Shephard (466) and Martindale (348) indicated it produces an ergogenic effect. Although caffeine may be purchased in powder or tablet form, it is a natural constituent of coffee, tea, kola nuts and cocoa beans. Preparations made from these plants contain varying amounts of caffeine; an eight-ounce cup of regular coffee may contain 150 mg, whereas tea and cola drinks may average approximately half as much. Some aspirin compounds contain 15 to 30 mg caffeine per tablet, while the various stay awake preparations contain approximately 110 mg/ tablet. A normal therapeutic dose of caffeine is 100 to 300 mg. For a brief, yet interesting, historical account of caffeine use, the reader is referred to *Drugs, Society and Human Behavior* (416).

Use in Athletics

The hypothetical beneficial use of caffeine as a doping agent in athletics is predicated on its action as a CNS stimulant, creating an increased alertness. This behavioral effect has been known empirically for centuries, and was recently resubstantiated experimentally in studies by Goldstein and his associates (211, 212). Physiologically, caffeine has increased urinary adrenalin secretion, possibly indicative of a stimulating effect on the adrenal medulla (325). If this could augment the natural release of adrenalin during exercise, it could possibly produce a potentiating effect.

Since caffeine is a natural ingredient of some common everyday beverages and foods, there is some controversy regarding its use in athletics; indeed, Ray (416) classifies caffeine as a "nondrug drug." Several reports (2, 309) have indicated that caffeine is commonly used in an attempt to increase athletic performance. However, Kourounakis (309) contended that in order to obtain an equivalent action to amphetamine, caffeine would have to be administered in a toxic dose. In 1939, Boje (56) stated the use of pure caffeine or preparations with a high caffeine content should be prohibited in connection with athletic competition. Yet he did indicate that coffee, tea or chocolate should not be forbidden altogether. More recently, Mustala (369) reported that caffeine was one of the few known drugs that may enhance athletic performance, and Kourounakis (309) would classify it as a doping agent. In 1962, the FISM undertook a study among Italian athletes, and reported that caffeine was one of the most used doping agents; subsequently, its use was forbidden in conjunction with athletic competition (518). However, the Medical Commission of the 1970 British Commonwealth Games did not regard caffeine, in the quantity normally found in a cup of coffee, as a doping agent. No evidence has been uncovered to indicate that it is banned by the NCAA, AAU, or IAAF. However, the statement relative to the use of any substance designed to facilitate performance may be interpreted to include caffeine. On the other hand, Fischbach (165) advocated the removal of caffeine from the doping list of the IOC and was successful in having it eliminated as a doping agent prior to the 1972 Olympics.

The problem relative to the use of caffeine in athletics is succinctly stated by Leake (318):

> There seems to be no public condemnation of the use of coffee by athletes, either before an athletic contest, or in ordinary living. Nevertheless, caffeine produces the same general sort of central stimulation and reduction of fatigue that is characteristic of the amphetamines, the only difference being that the effects of caffeine are commonly less than those of the amphetamines, and coffee is an anciently used and long established social beverage. No one seems ever to have raised the question about athletes taking a large drink of coffee before an athletic contest or game. In contrast to public indignation at the use of amphetamines to increase physical performance, the situation regarding caffeine is an interesting commentary on what constitutes social acceptability. It seems that what has long been used, what is well established in social custom, and about which people think they know the facts generally are sufficient to assure social acceptability.

What are the facts relative to caffeine and athletic performance?

Effects on Physical Working Capacity

Experiments with Animals

Using an *in vitro* preparation, Rudel (440) found that caffeine increased the force of muscular contraction in frog striated muscle fibers. The maximal force developed during tetanus can be increased by the addition of caffeine. Walther (532) tested the effect of caffeine upon an isolated nerve-muscle preparation (phrenic-diaphragm) and reported an increased efficiency upon muscle tissue that has been fatigued quickly as contrasted to muscle that has been fatigued over a longer period of time. Whether the results of these two experiments have any implications for human athletic performance would involve questionable extrapolation.

In more applied research, Jacob and Michaud (270) concluded that stimulating dosages of caffeine exerted no significant effect on swim time to exhaustion in mice. On the other hand, Villa and Panceri (529) found that high dosages of caffeine were effective in prolonging the run to exhaustion time of mice. Using four different groups of mice, they evaluated the effect of variant daily dosages (0, 0.1, 1.0, and 10.0 mg/kg) of caffeine upon run time to exhaustion. Their results indicated after 1 to 2 weeks, that the high dose level was effective, but the smaller dose levels did not appear to be.

It is obvious that the literature is limited relative to the physical performance of animals under the influence of caffeine, and that the results are contradictory. The dearth of animal research in this specific area may be due to the fact that caffeine is generally regarded as a harmless drug, and therefore, research as to its effect on athletic performance may be conducted safely with human subjects. However, it may be prudent for sportsmen, as well as other individuals, to limit their intake of coffee due to the positive statistical relationship between coffee consumption and coronary heart disease (396).

Experiments with Humans

The following review involves the effect of caffeine upon psychomotor performance tests and tests of strength and endurance, including local muscular endurance and general endurance.

Effect on Psychomotor Performance. As indicated in a previous section of this chapter, reaction time is one of the psychomotor abilities that has important implications for athletic success. The effect of caffeine on reaction time was first studied over sixty years ago. Hollingworth (253) reported small dosages (60-240 mg) impaired, whereas higher dosages (300-360 mg) appeared to decrease reaction time two hours after ingestion. Hawk (235) found that withdrawal from coffee drinking (2-6 cups/day) slowed reaction time, which could indicate caffeine had a beneficial effect. Cheney (92) reported simple reaction time was not affected by single doses of caffeine unless the dose exceeds 3.0 mg/kg. Higher dosages usually caused an impairment. In a subsequent study, Cheney (93) found that a caffeine alkaloid (3.3-3.6 mg/kg) and an equivalent amount of black coffee decreased reaction time on the order of 8 percent and 4 percent respectively. Thornton and his colleagues (506) indicated, in general, that 300 mg caffeine improved reaction time when compared with a control condition. In these older studies, methodological problems existed due to the lack of control over interfering variables which are known to affect reaction time.

In more recent studies with more sophisticated recording equipment and experimental methodology, results are controversial. Wenzel and Rutledge (538) used a rather intricate experimental design to study the influence of 0, 100, 200, and 300 mg caffeine upon several motor and psychomotor tests. In general, they noted caffeine induced a significant dose-related improvement in simple visual reaction time, but an inverse relationship was found between dose and effect on complex reaction time. Three hundred mg elicited a modest, although insignificant, decrease in performance. The authors concluded that if caffeine is to be used for the improvement of performance, at least in the simple tasks they used, then the dose should not exceed 100 mg. It is interesting to note that the average cup of coffee contains more than this dose. In an equally well-designed study, although also studying the effects of alcohol, Carpenter (85) found that three different caffeine dosages 0, 1.47, and 2.94 mg/kg), when interacting with zero dosages of alcohol, did not significantly affect simple reaction time. Lovingood and his coworkers (333) reported that 324 mg caffeine had no effect upon simple visual reaction time. In an effective review of the literature relative to the effect of caffeine upon motor control, Weiss and Laties (534) concluded the drug had little or no effect upon reaction time.

Although the last three reports indicate no significant effect of caffeine upon reaction time, the findings of Wenzel and Rutledge may warrant further investigation.

Effect on Strength and Endurance. The history of caffeine is full of empirical reports that it can increase work capacity. Catton, in *The Army of the Potomac,* noted that the coffee ration kept the Union army going. In a 1939 report from the Health Organization of the League of Nations, Boje (56) indicated that although there is no direct proof as to the beneficial effect of caffeine on athletic performance, it must be expected that its use as a doping agent is dangerous and therefore should be prohibited. However, general statements by Martindale (348) and Shephard (466) would appear to offer some evidence as to the effectiveness of caffeine. Martindale noted that caffeine facilitates the performance of muscular work and increases the total work which can be performed by a muscle. Shephard indicated caffeine can increase the capacity for physical exertion, as demonstrated by 20 to 30 percent more work output on a bicycle ergometer, increase aerobic power, and decrease the general sensation of fatigue. He also indicated caffeine compounds are undoubtedly taken by many endurance athletes, particularly long distance cyclists. On the other hand, Fischbach (164, 165) contended that normal doses will not affect athletes who are accustomed to coffee drinking, whereas high doses may cause a loss of sports performance ability. He also noted that normal doses may adversely affect those who are not accustomed to coffee.

A review of the literature would appear to indicate that the aforementioned comments by Martindale and Shephard are based upon *in vitro* studies and older research, as contemporary evidence does not substantiate these viewpoints. As discussed earlier, caffeine added to *in vitro* muscle preparations increased force, but these findings may not be applicable to the intact human organism. Moreover, analysis of the older studies, which follows below, ofttimes reveals erroneous generalizations due to methodological irregularities not known during the early era of drug experimentation with physical exertion in humans.

Alles and Feigen (14) indicated that as early as 1893, Mosso reported an increase in voluntary work capacity following the administration of small doses of caffeine. In 1907, using only two subjects (themselves) Rivers and Webber (428) reported an increased number and height of muscular contractions on a modified Mosso ergograph following the uptake of 300 mg caffeine citrate. They concluded caffeine increased the capacity for muscular work. In 1922, Herxheimer (244) noted caffeine did not affect performance of forty-six subjects in a 100 meter dash, but did increase work output on a bicycle ergometer task; he indicated, however, that no definite conclusions could be made due to the wide variability of the data. Further research was conducted immediately prior to and during World War II. It is difficult to interpret the results of Thornton and his associates (506), but they apparently concluded that 300 mg caffeine increases maximal grip strength as well as the muscular force level on a one-minute sustained isometric grip. With only three subjects (two males and one female), the interpretation is equivocal. Foltz and his associates (173) studied the effect of 500 mg caffeine sodium benzoate upon work output in a fatigued state. Four subjects performed a workload of 1235 kgm/minute to exhaustion and then received either a placebo or caffeine; the second ride to exhaustion was administered ten minutes later. Although the authors indicated that the caffeine facilitated recovery and subsequent performance on the second test, the interpretation is questionable since the conclusions were based on only two of the subjects. In a second study (174), 500 mg caffeine sodium benzoate was used to improve the working capacity of untrained subjects during bench stepping with a backpack, but the results were not conclusive as a training effect confounded the study. In a subsequent experiment with trained men (175), they noted a general improvement in work capacity on a bicycle ergometer. Alles and Feigen (14) reported no significant effect of 100, 200 or 400 mg caffeine upon work capacity under normal rested conditions. Haldi and Wynn (226) investigated the influence of 250 mg caffeine alkaloid upon a 100 yard swimming test for speed in twelve men; no beneficial or detrimental effect was found. Asmussen and Boje (26) studied the effect of 300 mg caffeine upon the ability of healthy athletes to perform two maximal work tasks on a bicycle ergometer; the work loads approximated energy expenditure in a 100 meter sprint and a 1500 meter run. Their results indicated that the ability of caffeine to stimulate the organism may overcome the inhibitory aspects of fatigue, especially in events of long duration. Lovingood and others (333) alluded to a study with Olympic athletes as subjects; caffeine was reported to enhance muscular performance in the high jump where mental precision is involved, but had no effect upon runners in the 100 yard dash, where speed was involved.

Based primarily upon a review of the above studies, Weiss and Laties (534) indicated that caffeine could prolong the amount of time an individual may perform physically exhausting work. More contemporary research would appear to contradict their statement. Ganslen and his colleagues (197), using five subjects, found that 200 mg had no effect upon work or aerobic capacity as determined by the Balke treadmill test. Margaria and others (341), administering 100 and 250 mg caffeine in five separate trials to three trained subjects, found no significant effect on maximal oxygen uptake or performance time on a treadmill run to exhaustion. Using twenty-five subjects, Bugyi (73) studied the effect of 167, 324 and 500 mg citrated caffeine upon the strength and endurance of the right forearm flexors; the workload consisted of maximal contractions at the rate of 30/minute for six minutes. The statistical analysis revealed all dosages had no effect on initial strength, final strength, fatigable work, or total work. The mathematical analysis of the rate of fatigue was similar under all conditions except the 500 mg dose, which pointed to a reduction in the overall rate of fatigue. In two separate experiments, Lovingood (331, 333) found isometric strength was unaffected by caffeine; dosages utilized were 324 and 500 mg citrated caffeine.

In summary, the effects of caffeine upon physical performance, especially involving prolonged exercise, appear to be open to question. Although more recent evidence indicates no effect of caffeine upon physical working capacity, the comments made relative to its effectiveness by such authorities as Shephard (466) and Weiss and Laties (534) should not be considered lightly.

NICOTINE

It may be rather unusual to consider smoking as an aid to athletic performance, but Kourounakis (309) would classify nicotine as a doping agent. Nicotine, a volatile alkaloid derived from tobacco, is present in the smoke of various tobacco preparations. A typical filter cigarette contains 20 to 30 mg nicotine, and the smoker who inhales will absorb approximately 10 per cent of this amount; experiments have indicated that one cigarette mimics the action of 1 mg nicotine injected intravenously (416). Although Silvette and his associates (471) indicated that the pharmacology of tobacco smoking and nicotine is not identical, they did note that doses of nicotine supplied in smoking can produce a pharmacological effect in man. However, other ingredients in smoke besides the nicotine may also elicit physiological effects. Nevertheless, smoking tobacco is an effective means of administering nicotine to the body. The interested reader is referred to Silvette and others (471) for a thorough discussion of nicotine pharmacology.

In general, small doses of nicotine act as a stimulant and affect the CNS and the sympathetic nervous system in a manner analogous to amphetamine. Ray (416) indicated it has no therapeutic action, but is used primarily to study synaptic functions. The possible use of nicotine as a doping agent in athletics may be due to its stimulating effect on the cerebral cortex (77) and the sympathetic ganglia (78, 324) as well as the ability to increase adrenalin secretion from the adrenal medulla (78, 205). Guyton (221) contended that nicotine does not directly affect the autonomic effector organ, but acts indirectly via its effect upon the hypothalamus. Larson and others (316) indicated nicotine may also elevate blood sugar levels, but that the effect is inconsistent in man. Thus, nicotine appears to be a sympathomimetic drug.

Other than experimentation with smoking, the literature is limited relative to the effect of nicotine upon human physical performance. This is understandable since nicotine is extremely toxic, with 60 mg constituting a lethal dose. Moreover, research as to the effect of smoking on physical performance, particularly of athletes, is also limited due to the hesitation of investigators to induce nonsmokers to smoke; in light of the statistical relationship between cigarette smoking and several pathological health conditions, this concern was and is warranted. Furthermore, most research which has been conducted in this area was primarily motivated because of the hypothetical adverse effects of smoking upon performance, and most studies involve comparisons of smokers and nonsmokers, or just involve the acute effects of smoking on various physiological or physical performance parameters in smokers alone.

In those experiments which used nicotine alone, the effects may be attributed to its pharmacological actions. However, in experimentation with smoking, it is difficult in most cases to determine whether the results are due to nicotine or to other substances present in the smoke. It has been shown, however, that smoking one cigarette will elicit the pharmacological actions of nicotine.

Effect of Smoking upon Physiological Adjustments to Exercise

Several investigators have noted detrimental effects of smoking on certain normal physiological adjustments to exercise. Nadel and Comroe (370) noted a decrease in airway conductance due to the acute inhalation of cigarette smoke; however, they did not attribute this effect to nicotine as it was filtered out. In a related context, Rode and Shephard (431) stated cigarette smoking appeared to increase the oxygen cost of breathing in near maximal exercise; a considerable percentual decrease in oxygen cost was noted when subjects abstained from smoking. Cooper (109) indicated smoking produced a decreased lung diffusing capacity during exercise, as well as a larger oxygen debt. Goldbarg and associates (208) found that smoking a single cigarette caused a higher heart rate and lower stroke volume during submaximal exercise, concluding that smoking decreased the efficiency of the heart. They noted the smaller stroke volume during exercise may be due to an added inotropic effect on the myocardium or decrease in venous return, despite the sympatho-mimetic effect caused by smoking. In a subsequent experiment (311), the decreased stroke volume was attributed to adverse effects of smoking upon peripheral venous return.

If the above physiological changes did occur during exercise as a result of smoking, they would appear to indicate deleterious effects upon athletic performance, particularly in events characterized by endurance. However, other investigators have noted no adverse effects of smoking on major physiological adjustments during exercise. Levy (327) and Schilpp (448) reported no significant effect of smoking on heart rate during exercise, while Henry and Fitzhenry (242) reported no effect upon oxygen consumption or oxygen debt in submaximal exercise.

Effect of Nicotine on Performance of Animals

The results of experimentation with nicotine and swimming performance of rats are about as divergent as possible. Using a swim test to exhaustion, Battig (44) reported nicotine in doses of 0.1 and 0.2 mg/kg improved the swimming endurance of rats. In a subsequent report (45), he found that four doses of nicotine (0.05, 0.1, 0.2, and 0.4 mg/kg) generally depressed performance levels; the swimming test consisted of ten trials for speed through a four meter water alley. The rats swam both with and without resistance. Regardless of the swimming condition, nicotine caused a considerable decrease in performance in the first two trials; results in trials 3 to 10 were inconsistent. Grandjean and Abelin (217) noted no influence of nicotine supplement upon the swimming performance of rats.

Effects of Smoking on Physical Working Capacity of Humans

In general, the available evidence indicated that the acute effect of smoking does not alter performance on a variety of physical performance tests. Using habitual smokers, Willgoose (540) indicated smoking caused a lower ability to recover from fatigue of the forearm flexor muscles and concluded athletes should refrain from nicotine during training. However, Kay and Karpovich (294) replicated his experiment and found no effect of smoking upon local muscular fatigue; they indicated Willgoose's results were the manifestation of a training or learning effect, since all nonsmoking trials were performed after the smoking trials. Anderson and Brown (18) resubstantiated the finding that smoking did not significantly alter grip strength or endurance. Using fifteen habitual smokers, Reeves and Morehouse (417) revealed smoking just prior to testing did not affect speed, strength, power or endurance. If the subject was a habitual smoker, no difference in performance was noted whether he abstained from smoking for several hours prior to performance or smoked up to the start of the event. In a similar study involving swimming performance, Pleasants and Grugan (404) reported that various periods of abstinence from smoking (15 minutes, 2 hours and 12 hours) had no significant effect upon 100 or 200 yard times of chronic smokers. Karpovich and Hale (289) evaluated the effects of cigarette smoking upon the ability to complete a standardized work load (48,928 foot pounds) on a bicycle ergometer. Although there was a trend towards better performance on nonsmoking days, the statistical analysis revealed no significant differences.

Although concrete conclusions relative to the effect of smoking, or nicotine, upon physical performance can not be derived from the available evidence, it would appear safe to assume that the acute effects are nil. That is to say, the smoking of several cigarettes just prior to performance will not enhance or deter physical performance. This is not to infer that chronic smoking patterns do not affect performance, particularly cardiorespiratory endurance capacity. If the aforementioned deleterious effects of smoking upon selected physiological adjustments to exercise are cumulative, then smoking would definitely limit aerobic capacity. With a little contemplation, one can realize the difficulty of designing a prospective study with the purpose of determining the effect of chronic smoking upon physical endurance in humans. Although retrospective studies (109) have noted greater cardiovascular endurance in nonsmokers as contrasted to smokers, there exist too many other interfering variables to attribute the difference solely to smoking.

PSYCHOTOMIMETIC DRUGS

A number of psychotomimetic (psychedelic or hallucinogenic) agents have become increasingly popular during the past two decades. Undoubtedly the most used psychotomimetic is marijuana, the active ingredient being a group of tetrahydrocannabinols; it is obtained from the dried mature flowering tops and leaves of a hemp plant, cannabis sativa. Hashish is the unadulterated resin exuded from the the hemp plant or dried flowers; it is derived from charas, the most potent cannabinol, and consequently is stronger than marijuana. Another popular hallucinogenic compound is lysergic acid diethylamide (LSD), a synthetic indole alkaloid derived from the ergot fungus claviceps purpurea. Although not an all-inclusive list, other psychedelic agents are mescaline, psilocybin, DOM (STP, 2:5 dimethoxy-4-methyl-amphetamine), and DMT (dimethyltryptamine).

The use of these agents elicits behavioral changes which may influence physical performance. Although they may produce subjective effects of euphoria, relaxation and a sense of well being, other effects may include alterations in cognition and perception distorting the individual's sense of time and space, changes in visual perception, and impaired immediate memory. Although there are some slight physiological changes associated with the social use of these drugs, they are primarily utilized for their psychological effects. The effects are dependent upon the type of drug, dosage, environment and personality of the user.

Very little research has been uncovered relative to the effect of psychotomimetic agents upon physical work capacity or athletic performance. Although one report (343) indicated marijuana affects primarily complex psychomotor tasks, Crancer and others (118) noted only slight effects upon simulated driving performance. In one of the only studies found testing the effects of hallucinogenic agents upon physical performance, Uyeno (514) noted that LSD had no effect on swimming speed of trained rats when compared to a saline control test.

With the limited evidence available, no conclusions may be made concerning the influence of psychotomimetic agents upon athletic performance. At present, the use of these agents is illegal; however, several groups are active in an attempt to legalize marijuana. Should legalization occur, it may precipitate research into the acute effects marijuana may exert upon physical performance. Since some have contended that marijuana may adversely affect the will power of the user, it may be wise for the athlete to abstain from its use during training; this reason for abstention is, of course, in addition to the legal implications.

CHAPTER 3

DRUGS AFFECTING THE NERVOUS SYSTEM—DEPRESSANTS

IN CONTRAST TO THE stimulants, depressants are drugs that decrease the activity of the CNS. They are used for a wide variety of reasons ranging from relief of minor pain to inducement of unconsciousness. Musser and O'Neill (367) classified CNS depressants in four categories: analgesics, sedatives and hypnotics, general anesthetics, and alcohol.

Analgesia represents the absence of sensibility to pain without loss of consciousness, and may be elicited by compounds ranging in potency from aspirin to morphine. Sedation and hypnosis represent varying degrees of depression; under sedation the subject may be completely cognizant of his environment and react to intellectual and motor tests in a normal manner although he is more tranquil, whereas hypnosis is a stronger depression usually characterized by sleep. Anesthesia represents a very strong depressive state with loss of feeling or sensation, especially pain. Although alcohol may fall into one of the above categories, it deserves an independent classification due to its common usage.

This method of classification is based upon the concept of therapeutic usefulness and does not represent a rigid categorization. Any one of the drugs in each category could be used to elicit either mild, moderate, or strong depression. Thus, under extreme dosages, aspirin could cause a state of anesthesia or even anesthetic death.

As is probably evident, hypnotics and anesthetics used to the point of inducing sleep have no practical value in athletics, except as a means of providing rest for the anxious athlete in the days prior to competition. However, all of the depressant drugs may be used in such a dosage as to produce a state of sedation and/or analgesia. The increased physical or psychical tolerance to pain may be a factor influencing resultant athletic performance.

As certain depressants may help to artificially improve the competitor's mental condition by modifying his reaction to pain, they fall under the definition of doping by the IAAF and IOC and are forbidden in conjunction with athletic competition. Under rule 144 of the IAAF, narcotic analgesics such as morphine, methadone, pethidine, dextromoramide, dipipanone and related compounds are currently proscribed. Although the rule makes no specific mention of other depressants such as barbiturates, major tranquilizers, or alcohol, these drugs may be covered by the general statement regarding doping, i.e. any substance which may improve performance. The IOC specifically proscribes tranquilizers, muscle relaxants, and ethyl alcohol, as well as narcotics such as morphine (309).

For the purpose of this discussion, the literature review was restricted to analgesics, sedatives, and alcohol, depressants which have been studied in relation to their effect upon physical performance. Although the literature concerning analgesics is limited, more extensive research has been conducted with tranquilizing agents and alcohol.

ANALGESIC DRUGS

Ikai and Steinhaus (264) have indicated that the perception of pain may be a limiting factor in the expression of muscular strength. Thus, any substance capable of reducing pain may increase performance capacity, as pain may be associated with extreme muscular effort. Analgesics are drugs which relieve pain. The interested reader is referred to Swerdlow (495) for an excellent discussion of analgesic pharmacology.

Mild Analgesics

Mild analgesics relieve pain without a sensation of drowsiness. The most common example is aspirin, or acetylsalicylic acid

(ASA), but other compounds such as phenacetin are also available. The exact mode of action of aspirin is obscure, although Collier (105) suggests the active ingredient, salicylate, may antagonize the action of bradykinin or other pain evoking substances. Aspirin is absorbed readily as acetylsalicylic acid, but is then hydrolyzed to salicylic acid. Salicylates are also antipyretic and may act directly upon the heat control mechanisms in the CNS with possible consequences for exercise in heat stress environments (144).

As an athlete may experience headache or other types of pain on a day of competition, aspirin may be recommended. Consequently, research has been conducted concerning its effect upon physical working capacity and various physiological adjustments during exercise. Downey and Darling (145) studied the action of acute (1½ hours prior to testing) and chronic (2-7 days prior to testing) ingestion of ASA on oxygen consumption during exercise. They found no evidence to indicate that salicylates affected exercise oxidative metabolism. In addition, exercise pulse rates were unaffected and no other significant cardiovascular changes were noted.

Fisher and his associates (166), using a double-blind placebo technique, studied the effect of aspirin (15 grains) on the max VO_2, maximal running time, and oxygen debt of nine highly trained collegiate cross country runners. No significant differences were noted for any of the criterion measures tested. However, the authors did note that not one subject complained of a headache during the test.

Aspirin causes a partial blocking of plasma FFA. Whitney and Ryan (539) hypothesized that this effect may be detrimental in endurance events, and subsequently conducted a controlled experiment to investigate the effects of normal aspirin dosage upon endurance performance. A double-blind placebo design was used, and the subjects injested either 0, 650, or 1300 mg ASA. Subjects were athletes in crew, track, and swimming, and they performed a sustained task indigenous to their sport. FFA levels were measured before and after the exercise task. The authors concluded aspirin did not impair the mobilization of FFA during exercise, nor did it have any influence upon the performance time in any of the events.

Several studies have investigated the effect of salicyclates upon physiological adjustments to exercise in the heat. Downey and Darling (144) indicated that acute and chronic ingestion of ASA had no effect on rectal temperature during rest, exercise, or recovery. Jacobson and Bass (272) tested the hypothesis that men given sodium salicylate would work in the heat at a lower temperature. Low doses had no effect upon skin or rectal temperature, pulse rate, and sweat rate. However, high dosages elicited a higher rectal temperature and sweat rate, findings contrary to their hypothesis. The same investigators (39) reported that the addition of sodium salicylate to an exercise regimen did not facilitate or hamper acclimatization to heat.

In summary, within the limitations of the research available, mild analgesics such as aspirin do not affect physical work capacity in normal or hot temperatures.

Potent Analgesics

The function of the more potent analgesics is to produce a stronger analgesic state. Codeine is more effective than aspirin, with morphine and its derivatives being among the most potent analgesics available. Morphine and other drugs such as heroin, methadone, pethidine, dextromoramide, and dipipanone are further classified as narcotics. The primary sites of action for morphine are the sensory cortex of the frontal lobe and the diencephalon (495) with depressive effects also upon the medulla and cerebellum (510).

Although the narcotic analgesics are proscribed by the IAAF and the IOC, there is little experimental evidence available to indicate that they do enhance athletic performance. They are probably banned due to their analgesic effects and possible ramifications for perception of pain during athletics. On the other hand, morphine may serve as an excitant to some individuals (495, 510); this effect may be similar to alcohol, acting by suppression of inhibitory mechanisms rather than by direct cortical stimulation.

In the only study uncovered testing the effects of strong analgesics upon work capacity, Jacob and Michaud (271) indicated morphine definitely prolonged the swim to exhaustion of mice. However, the mice were untrained and exposed to a water temperature of 20° C. The authors hypothesized that the beneficial effects of morphine in this case were due to its ability to reduce anxiety, since putting mice in water at 20° C does induce stress. Once the mice were trained in the swimming test, morphine had no effect on performance. Other analgesics (methadone, pethidine, dextromoramide and 3570 CT) had no significant effects upon performance, although causing slight motor problems in the mice.

One can readily understand the ethical problems involved concerning experimentation with narcotic analgesics in normal human athletes. However, if a definitive answer relative to their effect upon athletic performance is to be obtained, research under strict medical control needs to be conducted with humans. Whether or not such experimentation is necessary, or desirable, should be the joint consideration of the administrators and medical advisors of the various athletic governing bodies.

It is to be hoped that the athlete will have been educated to the potential hazards of narcotic analgesics.

SEDATIVE AGENTS—TRANQUILIZERS

Sedatives and hypnotics are often, pharmacologically, categorized together. Sedatives are agents that allay activity, tension, and excitement, whereas hypnotics are drugs utilized primarily to induce sleep. They act on various parts of the CNS. The classification of a drug as either a sedative or hypnotic is done primarily for therapeutic reasons, for usually drugs of this type may elicit either sedative or hypnotic effects. Barbiturates are primarily classified as hypnotics, but in the appropriate dose have been utilized as sedatives. The major and minor tranquilizers are sedative in nature, and have broad therapeutic application in the medical field.

The primary major tranquilizers in use today are synthetically produced phenothiazines; chlorpromazine is a drug in this class, and brand names include Compazine®, Thorazine®, Sparine®, and others. The rauwolfia alkaloids, primarily reserpine, are also classified as major tranquilizers. The major tranquilizers include the butyrophenones, thioxanthenes, and piperioine and piperazine side chain compounds. As a class, the major tranquilizing drugs are powerful antipsychotic agents and are used primarily to control severe mental disturbances. Their use for common nervous tension is contraindicated (205).

The minor tranquilizers are more commonly used, allaying simple anxiety, tension, insomnia, and restlessness. Barbiturates had been used previously for these purposes, but they have been replaced by such compounds as meprobamate (Miltown® or Equanil®), a substituted idol, and chlordiazepoxide (Librium®), a benzodiazephine. Other general classes of minor tranquilizers include the thiazole and diphenylmethane derivatives.

Use in Athletics

The rationale for the use of tranquilizing agents in athletics is obscure. In 1939, Boje (56) did not classify tranquilizing substances as doping since there appeared to be no danger of abuse among athletes; he indicated the drugs are mainly fatigue producing rather than fatigue alleviating. However, they were on the list of proscribed doping agents for the 1972 Olympic Games.

The use of tranquilizers may be effective in reducing pre-competition tension. Ryde (443), discussing the athlete's nervous system, contended that although experience helps to reduce stress, some international level athletes are still jittery before competition. Thus, while Boje (56) indicated there was little danger of these drugs being abused in athletics, he did concede that the use of tranquilizers to relieve nervous disturbances prior to competition may enable the athlete to attain a higher performance level.

Murphy (364) stated that although the extensive use of sedatives in athletics is to be condemned, the use of meprobamate or phenobarbitol in the athlete who is over-keyed for a game may be beneficial in helping him perform normally. However, Buterbaugh (81) cautioned the athlete on use of these agents. Since most of the tranquilizers such as Miltown, Equanil, and Librium cause some degree of sedation, the response of the athlete may be opposite to that desired, i.e. he may become too sedated with an adverse effect upon his physical performance.

It would appear that the main rationale against the use of tranquilizers in athletics is their beneficial effect upon pre-competition tension. This tranquilizing effect may be extremely important in riflery, archery, figure skating, and other activities where the tension may have a detrimental effect on performance.

As an interesting side point, deVries and Adams (135) noted that fifteen minutes of low intensity exercise may produce greater neuromuscular relaxation than 400 mg meprobamate.

On the other hand, there may be other effects of tranquilizers which may benefit performance. Chlorpromazine and other major tranquilizers may alter the individual's reaction to pain by induc-ing a state of emotional indifference, thus enabling an athlete to go beyond his natural limits. Moreover, Root and Hoffmann (436) indicate there are two pharmacological and behavioral phases to the action of resperpine. In the first short phase, amines are liberated and elicit the peripheral symptoms of the sympathomimetics; the catecholamine level of the blood is increased; Adamson and Finley (5) noted a psychostimulant effect with small doses of oxypertine. The second longer phase is characterized by peripheral parasympathetic effects and sub-sequent relaxation. If the athlete performed while in the first phase, the effect of reserpine would be analogous to amphetamine.

Some tranquilizers also serve as potent vasodilators, especially rauwolfia and the veratrum alkaloids. The effects of vasodilators on performance is considered in Chapter 5.

Experiments with Animals

LeBlanc (320) tested the effect of 10 mg/kg chlorpromazine upon the endurance swimming capacity of rats. The water temperature appeared to be an interacting factor for chlorpro-mazine adversely affected the swimming performance at 19°

and 28° C, but had no influence at 32° C. Jacob and Michaud (269) found that low doses of meprobamate increased the swim to exhaustion time in mice. In a subsequent report (270) they concluded central sedation by meprobamate with adequate dosages and time schedule may prolong the swim time to exhaustion. However, heavy sedation by either meprobamate or hexobarbital shortens the swim time. Utilizing a swimming test for speed, Kleinrok and Swiezynska (301) found that reserpine (0.3 mg/kg) increased swimming speed in unweighted rats, but had no effect on the speed of rats with weights attached to their tails. Using three racehorses in a series of runs, Stewart (492) noted a statistically significant decrease in speed following the administration of 0.5 mg/kg promazine.

The effectiveness of tranquilizing agents upon the work capacity of animals appears to be contradictory, but the report from Jacob and Michaud (270) may indicate the effect is dose dependent.

Experiments with Humans

Subjective Effects

As one of the hypothetical reasons for using tranquilizers as doping agents is their effect upon anxiety and tension, it would be informative to study behavioral and mood changes following ingestion. Policreti and his associates (406) concluded, within the restriction of a small number of subjects, that not only stimulant agents but depressants such as Librium exert a favorable influence upon the attentive ability of athletes. Adamson and Finley (5) noted that oxypertine, although a tranquilizing agent at high dose levels, may have stimulant properties at lower dosages. Dosages of five and ten mg were found to produce a definite enhancement in the mood of five trained athletes, whereas larger dosages (20 and 40 mg) did not. Similar findings were reported by Smith and Beecher (480) although different subjects were used in the groups receiving different dosages. In the fifteen swimmers who received 100 mg secobarbital, moods and physical states were characterized by intoxication, elation, and deactivation; the authors indicated these changes would appear to hinder performance. Moreover, the swimmers experienced distortion in judgement (481). Although the performer perceived his performance as being faster under the influence of secobarbital, the drug condition was actually slower than control. Thirty-eight throwers and runners received 50 mg secobarbital. The reported general effect of this dosage was one of physical elation and activation, effects also elicited by the amphetamine dosages used in their study.

Thus, in summary, tranquilizing or sedative agents given in certain dosages may produce behavioral and mood changes analogous to amphetamines, or may also produce a state of relaxation.

Effect on Reaction Time

Several investigators have reported a slower reaction time due to tranquilizers, but the majority of reports indicate no significant effect of small dosages. Kornetsky (306) indicated that 1600 mg meprobamate significantly impaired reaction time while neither 800 mg meprobamate nor 60 mg and 120 mg phenobarbital had any effect. Reitan (419) administered a battery of psychological tests, including simple and discrimination reaction time, for the purpose of studying the comparative effects of placebo, ultran, and meprobamate under standardized conditions. He administered 1200 mg meprobamate two hours prior to testing, and an additional 400 mg one hour prior; ultran was given in 900 and 300 mg respectively. Considering all eight tests as a unitary criterion score, Reitan concluded that the placebo produced significantly better results than either of the two tranquilizers. In a follow up study in the same report, sixteen subjects consumed 400 mg of the same drugs four times a day for six days prior to testing on the same battery of tests. In this study, no significant differences were noted on any of the tests.

Frankenhaeuser and Myrsten (182) studied the effect of 800 mg meprobamate upon choice-reaction tasks of varying difficulty. The results indicated that the meprobamate impaired performance on the more difficult tasks, whereas little difference existed between placebo and drug conditions with the smaller doses.

Of equal importance in this study was the fact that the higher the learning level of the subject to the task, the less the effect of the drug. Thus, motor skills which are overlearned, which is the case in most skilled athletes, may not be adversely affected by tranquilizers. In a complex study, Wenzel and Rutledge (538) evaluated the effect of four tranquilizers upon simple visual and choice reaction times; drugs and dosages included phenobarbital (15, 30, and 45 mg), chlorpromazine (25, 50, and 100 mg), meprobamate (200, 400, and 800 mg), and oxanamide (200, 400, and 800 mg). None of the drugs had any effect on either reaction time test.

Using a double-blind placebo study, Rasch and his colleagues (415) studied the effect of 800 mg meprobamate upon simple visual reaction time and movement time. The drug was administered two hours prior to testing. The authors concluded that meprobamate, in the commonly used dosage associated with competitive athletics, had no effect upon either parameter tested. Using trained athletes, Adamson and Finley (5) reported no effect of oxypertine (0, 5, 10, 20, and 40 mg) upon reaction time.

In no studies did tranquilizers facilitate reaction time. The impairment effect appears to be dependent upon dosage and complexity of the reaction time test. High dosages produce a slower reaction time in more complex tasks, whereas small doses appear to have little or no effect.

Effect on Physiological Adjustments to Exercise

The effect of a particular tranquilizer upon the physiological adjustment to exercise may be primarily dependent upon pharmacological effects other than its tranquilizing action. For example, tranquilizers are used as antihypertensive agents and consequently may have profound effects upon the cardiovascular-respiratory system. According to Krumholz and Ross (312), reserpine depletes norepinephrine and causes a peripheral vasodilation; reserpine therapy (0.5 mg/day for 7 days) has been shown to decrease pulmonary diffusing capacity.

Chlorthiazide, in addition to being an antihypertensive agent, is also diuretic. In a controlled study, Danzinger and Cumming

(128) noted that after three days of chlorthiazide ingestion (1.5 g daily), normal subjects experienced a 21 percent fall in plasma volume and a concomitant decrease in physical working capacity (15%) and max VO_2 (11%). In this case, the impaired physiological adjustments would be attributed to the diuretic effect on plasma volume, and not any tranquilizing effect *per se.*

Bruce and his associates (71) studied the effect of chemical antihypertensives (chlorthiazide, reserpine, methyl dopa and clonidine) upon maximal oxygen uptake levels in sixteen patients with essential hypertension and fifty slightly younger asymptomatic Negro male workers with high blood pressure. At the end of the six month treatment program, the antihypertensive therapy produced a statistically significant increase in the maximal oxygen uptake and treadmill endurance times of the patients, but had no effect on the workers. Chidsey and others (96) evaluated the effects of large parenteral doses of a rauwolfia alkaloid (syrosingopine) upon various cardiovascular parameters during exercise (1500 foot pounds/minute on a bicycle ergometer). Although the pulse rate showed a consistent reduction after injection of the drug, cardiac output was unaffected during exercise. Ganslen and others (197) noted that Equanil taken in 400 mg doses five times daily, or in single dosages of varying amounts up to 800 mg, had no effect upon the cardiovascular response to the Balke treadmill test of aerobic capacity. At large dosages (1200 mg), the authors hypothesized a depressant effect upon cardiac output. In support of this hypothesis Carlsson and associates (84), although using patients, indicated that large doses of chlorpromazine usually resulted in a lower stroke volume and relatively low cardiac output during work on a bicycle ergometer.

Although a plethora of literature exists relative to the physiological effects of tranquilizers during rest, only a few studies were uncovered evaluating their action during exercise. Consequently, no sound conclusions may be made concerning the influence of tranquilizing agents upon the cardiovascular, respiratory, and metabolic adjustments to exercise, although it appears large doses may be detrimental to factors associated with endurance.

*Effect on **Human Performance**—Laboratory Experimentation*

Several investigators have studied the effects of tranquilizers upon strength and local muscular endurance. Costello (113) determined the maximum strength of his subjects on a hand dynamometer and then instructed them to maintain two thirds of this strength level as long as possible. Meprobamate (800 mg) and Seconal® (3 gr) had no significant effect in contrast to a placebo and no drug condition. Using the same design with women subjects, the tranquilizers again did not increase or decrease endurance. Adamson and Finley (5) reported that small dosages of oxypertine (5 and 10 mg) had no significant effect upon a group of isometric strength tests or an isotonic endurance test, but large dosages (20 and 40 mg) impaired muscular strength. In general, the results indicated a decrement in isometric strength with increasing dosages, but no influence upon isotonic endurance. Bujas and others (75) indicated that Veronol® (diethylbarbituric acid) exerted no effect on an arm hang for endurance in subjects who were rested and motivated.

Only a few studies have been found that investigated the effect of tranquilizers upon general endurance capacity. Borg and his associates (58) studied the influence of 300 mg amobarbital upon performance during a bicycle ergometer strength and endurance test. The amobarbital caused a general decrease in endurance capacity, and the authors concluded this result was primarily due to the psychopharmacological effect of decreased motivation for work. Ganslen and others (197) found no effect of small doses of Equanil (up to 800 mg) upon performance on the Balke treadmill test, but did note that large doses elicited a general disinclination to work during the early stages of the treadmill test. Bujas and others (75) reported that diethylbarbituric acid had no effect upon a bicycle ergometer ride or treadmill run for endurance.

In summary, although the tranquilizing or sedative drugs may produce a sensation of elation and activation, as discussed previously, they do not appear to produce positive results on tests involving muscular strength or local muscular general endurance. If anything, the literature suggests a detrimental effect, particularly with high doses. The following section corroborates this general statement.

Effect on Human Performance—Field Tests

Although primarily investigating the effects of amphetamines upon athlete performance, Smith and Beecher (479, 480, 481) utilized secobarbital as a treatment in order to mask the subjective effects of the amphetamines. Secobarbital was used in five of the six separate experiments. In the first experiment, 100 mg secobarbital was administered to fifteen swimmers; 50 mg was utilized in three experiments with runners and one experiment with weight throwers and shot putters. The 100 mg dose significantly impaired the performance in the swimmers, but the 50 mg dose had no effect upon the other groups. However, the experimental design and conduct of the study had some serious limitations; the reader is referred to Chapter 2 concerning amphetamines and human performance—field experimentation.

ALCOHOL

Alcohol is a drug. Beverages containing ethyl alcohol, or ethanol, are consumed by the majority of the adult population throughout the world, and although the vast majority are social drinkers, a considerable number of individuals abuse the use of alcohol. Indeed, alcohol is the number one drug problem in the United States both in the adult and teenage populations (12). Although the chronic ingestion of alcohol leading to addiction and alcoholism is an important problem, with implications for physical fitness, it falls outside the scope of this book. Thus this section will deal with the acute effects of alcohol ingestion upon physical performance.

Ethyl alcohol is not a foreign substance to the body, as it can be isolated in small amounts from any animal tissue or organ (391). Although exogenous sources of alcohol may be taken into the body in a variety of ways, the oral route is the most common. It is absorbed directly from the stomach and small intestine into the blood stream, with maximum concentration occurring in less than one hour. Alcohol is distributed in the water of the body, and its concentration in each tissue depends upon the water content of that tissue. Thus, the distribution of alcohol in the body is essentially a process of dilution. The elimination of alcohol proceeds at a constant rate, approximately three quarters of an ounce per hour. It is oxidized in three stages, with the first rate-limiting stage occurring primarily in the liver; alcohol dehydrogenase converts alcohol to acetaldehyde. The acetaldehyde is transformed to acetic acid, which is subsequently oxidized to carbon dioxide and water. In the process, one gram of alcohol yields seven calories.

The alcohol content in the body may be detected through blood analysis, although the Breathalyzer is commonly used by law enforcement agencies. Blood alcohol levels (BAL) are expressed in milligrams (mg) per 100 milliliters (ml) of blood. Thus, a BAL of 40 mg/100 ml blood would be expressed as .04 percent or 40 mg percent. BAL's up to .05 percent are not usually intoxicating, and the effect above the .05 level is dependent upon the individual. Many states interpret the .10 level as being legally intoxicated, whereas at the .15 to .20 level, most individuals are definitely drunk.

Use in Athletics

Alcohol affects all cells of the body, the most dramatic results of ingestion being the effects on the brain. Gould (213) indicated that in spite of the long use of alcohol as a stimulant, it is actually a central nervous system depressant. The apparent stimulation is evinced because of the depressive action of ethanol on the reticular activating system. The inhibitory control mechanisms are decreased and this results in unrestrained activity of many areas of the brain with loss of the integrating control of the cerebral cortex. Several investigators (140, 399) have noted a stimulation effect of alcohol in some individuals, but attributed the cause to increased secretions from the adrenal medulla and increased sympathetic nervous activity. A biphasic hypothesis regarding the effects of alcohol has been advanced, indicating that it may produce a transitory sensation of excitement followed by depressive effects. Thus, the application of alcohol may be based upon two paradoxical effects. In some cases, it may be used for the apparent stimulating effect, while in others for the depressive or tranquilizing effect on reducing excessive tension.

Boje (56) and Wolf (552) indicated that in cases of extreme athletic exertion, or in events of brief maximal effort, alcohol has been given to athletes to serve as a stimulant by releasing inhibitions and lessening the sense of fatigue. This viewpoint relative to mental stimulation, which has been reiterated by others (94, 223, 247, 264, 273), would suggest alcohol exerts its influence through its effects on the subject's state of the mind. As an illustration, Jokl (279) reported evidence that alcohol was in wide use in European athletics at the turn of this century. He reported cases of a cyclist imbibing rum and champagne throughout a 24-hour race, jockeys pouring champagne down the throats of their horses before the race, and marathon runners and walkers consuming considerable quantities of cognac or beer during competition. Rationale for their use was ascribed to their refreshing effect or the ability to restore the athlete's strength. On the other hand, Shephard (466) noted that in some events, anxiety may disrupt performance by inducing excessive arousal of the cerebral cortex. In this case, the sedative action of alcohol may be beneficial. Marty Liquori, one of the top milers in the United States, reportedly consumes several beers the night before competition in order to relax and have sound sleep.

Although alcohol is a common beverage, and is part of the normal menu in several European countries, Ulmark (512) indicated that alcohol should be forbidden to all athletes in training and during competition. It was proscribed as a doping agent by the IOC, and Shephard (466) noted that two pistol-shooters were disqualified during the 1968 Olympics due to the alleged use of alcohol in an attempt to increase their competitive ability. Fischbach (165), however, noted that alcohol, although called goldwater by athletes involved in shooting competition, was not listed as a specific doping agent for the 1972 Munich Olympics.

Since alcohol is a popular beverage with potent pharmacological effects on behavior, it has received considerable research attention in relationship to physical performance. The majority of the research has centered about psychomotor ability, primarily in skills involving automobile operation, but a considerable number of studies also have been conducted regarding its influence upon intense muscular effort.

Experimentation with Humans

Subjective Effects

An abundance of studies have been conducted in order to document the effect of alcohol on psychological processes. A number of these have dealt with the acute effects of intoxication, but they are not pertinent to this discussion as it is highly unlikely that an athlete would become intoxicated just prior to an event. Coopersmith (110) succinctly summarized current knowledge regarding the effect of small amounts of alcohol upon behavior in normal subjects. He noted both popular impressions and the clinical and anthropological evidence suggest that alcohol reduces feelings of insecurity, tension and discomfort, and thereby permits a freer and less constrained behavioral expression. Thus, as Shephard (466) has noted, alcohol may elicit greater self-confidence in the athlete.

These statements reinforce the concept, advanced in the preceding section, that the acute ingestion of small amounts of alcohol may be ergogenic in nature due to inhibition of psychological factors which may limit performance.

Effects on Psychomotor Performance

Sollman (486) stated that the physical symptoms of ethanol ingestion show individual differences according to temperament and circumstances, but with increasing doses they tend to run a descending course on a continuum from euphoria to coma. Motor symptoms follow a similar, but not necessarily parallel, course.

Extensive research has been conducted relative to the effect of alcohol on psychomotor performance, especially in the realm of driver skills. No comprehensive coverage of these studies is offered here, since it falls outside the scope of this presentation, and Carpenter (86) has succinctly summarized the findings. In a critical review of studies from 1940 to 1961 concerning the effects of alcohol on some psychological processes, including reaction time, Carpenter has noted in general that motor performance is impaired at low and moderate blood alcohol levels. In a series of tests during the same time period, Hebbelinck (238) also noted in tests of physical performance that neuromuscular performance was adversely affected at BAL's lower than .05; he later concluded that neuromuscular incoordination and poorer reflexive control appeared to be responsible mainly for the deteriorative effects of alcohol on the basic components of physical performance (240). Nelson (377) reiterated these viewpoints, indicating that highly coordinated skills seemed to decrease most in efficiency following alcohol injection. He observed deteriorative effects of two and three ounces of pure ethanol upon reaction time and accuracy.

More recent investigations substantiate the fact that psychomotor performance is retarded at low blood alcohol levels. Significant decrements in hand-eye coordination (467), balance (49), complex coordination (498), and visual tracking (176) have been reported at BAL's between .04 to .06.

Summarizing a number of laboratory reports, Shephard (466) noted a variety of measures such as arm steadiness, body sway, dynamic balance, and more complicated psychomotor tests are all adversely affected by alcohol, even as low as 30 mg/100 ml; all subjects show a loss of motor performance at 100 mg/100 ml.

In summary, the evidence overwhelmingly supports the conclusion that alcohol does adversely affect fine psychomotor performance. However, Shephard (466) interjects the intriguing thought that the greater self-confidence produced by alcohol may override the loss of skill and slowing of body reactions.

Effect on Physiological Adjustments to Exercise

The effect of alcohol upon cardiovascular, respiratory,, and metabolic adjustments to submaximal and maximal exercise has been investigated recently. Heart rate response has received considerable attention. Studies concerning the effect of alcohol on the resting heart rate appear to be contradictory. Several investigators (219, 236, 282, 292, 425) have noted an increase following the administration of ethanol, while others (140, 199, 213, 287, 537) revealed no effect. Hebbelinck (236) evaluated the effect of a moderate dose (0.6 ml/kg) of absolute alcohol on the cardiac response before, during, and after a five minute workload at 1500 kpm. He noted an increase of four systoles per minute during rest and recovery, and a marked average increase of twenty-three beats per minute during the early stages of the workload. In a subsequent report (239), using a small dose of ethanol and a workload of 1000 kpm, identical results were obtained. Although his data are indicative of a significant cardiac response, no statistical analyses were performed. Adolph (6) found that the ingestion of 1 ml/kg pure ethanol produced a statistically significant tachycardia during the first five minutes of the Balke treadmill test. However, of the six subjects, two had resting heart rates during the alcohol phase which averaged thirty beats higher than the control phase, a finding which may influence the results as previous research (543) has indicated a high relationship between the resting heart rate and the initial stages of a submaximal work task. Blomqvist and colleagues (52) reported that 150 ml of 86 proof alcohol elevated the heart rate 12 to 14 beats per minute during submaximal exercise. The rate during maximal exercise was unchanged. However, they did not counterbalance the order of treatments in this repeated-measure design. Furthermore, the control study, which involved a maximal workload, was conducted on the same day two hours prior to the experimental phase. Thus, as noted by the authors, the conclusions might be influenced by the fact that previous research (234) has indicated a relative increase in the heart rate response during light submaximal workload if preceded by exercise at a heavier workload.

Contrary to the above, other studies indicate alcohol exerts no effect on cardiac response to exercise. Mazess and others (351), using 0.6 g ethanol/kg and a workload of 1000 kpm, found no significant differences in heart rate before, during, and after work at sea level; but, they did note a detrimental effect at altitude. Using three different types of work (step-wise increases, continuous, and intermittent), Garlind and associates (200) found that the average heart rate response to submaximal work tests was not influenced significantly by ethanol. However, investigation of the report revealed several problems which could prejudice the interpretation of this data. In addition, marked differences were noted in several of the individual scores and yet no statistical analysis was undertaken. Riff and colleagues (425) found no effect of ethanol (6 oz. of 90 proof Bourbon) on the hemodynamic response to a five-minute workload of 600 kpm. Using four different dosages of pure ethanol (0.0, 0.2, 0.4, and 0.6 ml/lb), Bobo (54) revealed no change in exercise heart rate at submaximal or near maximal runs on a treadmill. Williams (545) concluded that three variant dosages (0.0, 0.2, 0.4 ml/lb) had no significant effect on heart rate response to exercise at 500, 1000, 1500 kpm on a bicycle ergometer. In a subsequent study (547), a moderate dose (0.4 ml/lb) had no effect on either submaximal heart rate (400-1200 kpm) or maximal heart rate determined just prior to exhaustion on an all-out bicycle ride.

The available evidence would appear to support the conclusion that alcohol exerts little or no influence upon the heart rate response to exercise, particularly during maximal work. The mass sympathetic discharge to the heart during exercise would appear to override the theoretical adrenergic effect of alcohol postulated by Perman (399).

Gould (213) reported that alcohol may serve as a myocardial depressant in man, decreasing cardiac output without a change in heart rate. Summarizing other investigations with animals, he indicated that alcohol reduced cardiac contractility. However, it is not known whether these results may be extrapolated to man during exercise. The findings of Blomqvist (52) indicated no influence of ethanol on cardiac contractility during exercise since maximal cardiac output and stroke volume did not change.

One of the physiological effects of ethanol during rest is a cutaneous vasodilation, with a concomitant vasoconstriction in resting musculature (162, 214). If this condition persisted during exercise, it could prove detrimental if the cardiac output did not compensate. However, Graf and Strom (214), using venous occlusion plethysmography to study skin and muscle blood flow, reported that ethanol did not measurably influence the central circulatory response to leg work and did not decrease physical work capacity.

Garlind and his associates (200) reported that neither a small (0.3 g/kg) nor a moderate dose (0.6 g/kg) of absolute alcohol had any effect upon the respiratory rate, respiratory quotient, ventilatory quotient, or oxygen uptake in nine subjects before, during, or after exercise. In other reports concerning oxygen consumption, Blomqvist and others (52) found that oxygen uptake during submaximal work was 0.05 to 0.15 L/minute higher after administration of alcohol. Adolph (6) also reported small, but not significant, increases in oxygen uptake during the early stages of the Balke treadmill test following alcohol ingestion. Conversely, Mazess (351) found no significant effect during submaximal work while Bobo (54) reported similar findings for both submaximal and near maximal exercise with four dosage levels of alcohol. Williams (545) also reported no significant effect of a small or moderate dose upon oxygen consumption during submaximal and near maximal exercise on a bicycle ergometer; also, no changes were noted in oxygen uptake during a five minute recovery period. In general, these studies indicate that alcohol has no effect on maximal oxygen consumption capacity.

In summary, it would appear that the acute ingestion of ethanol elicits neither favorable nor unfavorable physiological modifications in the cardiovascular, respiratory, or metabolic responses to exercise, particularly if it is maximal exercise. Apparently the various physiological changes produced by alcohol during a resting state are abrogated by the various neural and hormonal adjustments associated with the onset of exercise.

Effect on Strength and Endurance—Laboratory Experiments

Since alcohol has been a common beverage for thousands of years, and its behavioral effects well-known by medical personnel, it was one of the first substances investigated regarding its ergogenic effect. Most of the early research dealt with its effect upon local muscular strength and fatigue, while later studies included tests of general endurance capacity.

The first recorded experiments concerning the effects of alcohol on muscular fatigue were reported by Lombard (330) in 1892. He utilized the ergograph designed by Mosso to measure the effect of alcohol on the flexor muscles of the second finger. Only limited data were obtained with small doses involving one subject. The quantities taken greatly increased the endurance of voluntary muscular power, at least within the limited scope of this study. Lombard attributed the increase to the effect of alcohol on the CNS.

A comprehensive review of the literature published prior to 1908 was presented by Rivers (427). As in Lombard's study, several irregularities can be noted in the experimental methodology. For example, only one or two subjects were used, with general conclusions based on their performances. Also, in the majority of studies, no mention was made of such factors as control doses, assignment of dose by body weight, presence of food in the digestive tract, or the type of alcohol administered, all of which are considered today to bear upon the acceptability of the results. However, it would not be proper to criticize these early investigators, for some of the fine points of experimental design in alcohol studies were unknown at that time. Nevertheless, these limitations should be considered when interpreting the results of the early research.

Rivers (427) noted that the work of Hellsten was the most extensive done at that time, and indicated it was the only work which clearly illustrated the deleterious influence of alcohol on the capacity for muscular work. Using an ergograph to test endurance, Hellsten took 25 to 30 grams of absolute alcohol approximately five to ten minutes before beginning muscular work and found that the daily effect was so slight that differences might be due to chance variation. However, at a dose of eighty grams he found a distinct deleterious effect. In another series of experiments, Hellsten tested the effects of alcohol taken at different intervals before beginning to perform muscular work immediately after ingestion, thirty minutes, one hour, and two hours later. In all cases, alcohol diminished the amount of work done; the results refer to the total amount of work done during twenty short ergographic bouts, but when the alcohol was taken immediately prior to the beginning of work, there was an initial increase in work output. This finding may represent the first evidence in support of the biphasic hypothesis, an initial stimulating sensation followed by depressive action.

Rivers (427) also cited the work of Joteyko concerning the effect of alcohol on muscular fatigue. Using ergographic methods, she found that with contractions every six or eight seconds, alcohol may prevent the occurrence of fatigue. With a rhythm of six seconds fatigue was elicited in fifteen minutes, but after a dose of twenty grams of alcohol, there was no evidence of fatigue after one hour. Partridge (395), using a dynamometer, measured six sets of one hundred contractions each, given at the rate of one every 1.6 seconds, in one hour. In one subject, he found that a dose of twenty grams of absolute alcohol produced a decrease in power, while in another individual, doses of fifteen and thirty grams had no effect on the total amount of work done.

Not all of the early studies reviewed by Rivers (427) were included in this discussion; only a few examples were cited. However, the following was River's general summarizing statement in 1908:

> The results of this historical survey may be summarized as follows: Nearly all who have used the ergograph in their investigations have found that alcohol increases the capacity for work either under certain conditions, or in certain persons, or for a certain time. When we turn to the details of the mode of action of alcohol on the ergographic curve, we find that the majority of those who consider the point find that the effect of alcohol is chiefly on the number of contractions.

However, in a series of experiments on himself and another subject, Rivers (427) failed to confirm the conclusions of nearly all previous workers that small doses of alcohol, from five to twenty ml, had an immediate stimulatory or depressant action on the capacity for muscular work as tested on the ergograph. He continued to state that the results of most of those who found the capacity for muscular work increased under the influence of small doses have been due, not to the physiological action of the substances, but to the interest aroused by taking the alcohol and the sensory stimulation involved in swallowing it. Those who have found a diminution in the amount of work must be open to the charge of having been influenced by suggestion. Thus, he attributes previous results to psychological reasons.

Rivers, whose experiments involved more adquate experimental control, but whose statistical inferences are open to question, found evidence that a small dose neither increased nor decreased the capacity for muscular work. With a large dose, forty ml absolute alcohol, he cited evidence in one case of an increase in the amount of work, but the increase was not systematic.

In more recent years, several reports have resubstantiated the conclusions of Rivers. Hebbelinck (236) reported no significant effect of 0.6 ml/kg absolute alcohol upon muscular strength; however, he did report a slight decrease in power. In a subsequent study (240), although several individuals did better on strength and power tests under the influence of alcohol, he concluded that static strength as measured by a manuometer and back dynamometer was not changed after consumption of a small dose of alcohol. On the other hand, dynamic strength showed a decrease of 5.8 percent.

Contrary to Hebbelinck's findings, Nelson (377) indicated that two and three ounces of pure alcohol elicited a decrease in isometric grip strength. Of the various gross motor tests involved in his study, he concluded strength was one of the most adversely affected. Jellinek (273) reported a 10 percent decrease in ergographic muscular output from the effects of one to three ounces of alcohol.

In an experiment to measure the effect of alcohol on several parameters, Simonson and Ballard (472) reported that the effects of alcohol on muscle strength were inconclusive. Testing subjects at five time intervals, ranging from fifteen minutes to three hours after ingestion of alcohol, they noted no constant effects upon the strength of the hand and arm extensor muscles. In a comprehensive coverage of neurological and physiological studies with alcohol, Pihkanen (401) alluded briefly to a dynamometer strength test on nine subjects, who on three occasions received either beer, an alcohol solution, or an equivalent amount of water; the findings indicated only a slight impairment of performance after being compared to the water series. However, he conjectured that this was an effect of psychic fatigue. In a well-controlled study, Ikai and Steinhaus (264) evaluated the effect of alcohol on measured tension in the right forearm flexors, using one maximum contraction per minute for thirty minutes. Ten subjects were used in a blank control series in order to establish a curve of fatigue, and were observed again in five maximum pulls before the consumption of 15 to 20 ml of 95 percent ethyl alcohol in water. Two minutes after the alcohol was taken, testing was continued once a minute for twenty-five minutes. For each session, all contractions recorded after alcohol consumption were averaged. The mean of the ten averages after alcohol was compared with the mean of the ten averages of the adjusted blank control performances of the same ten subjects. An increase of 3.7 pounds, or 5.6 percent, was attributable to alcohol. However, this increase was not statistically significant.

Williams (542) studied the interaction effects of a control (0.0 ml/lb), small (0.2 ml/lb), moderate (0.4 ml/lb), and large (0.6 ml/lb) dose of alcohol with variant elapsed time periods following ingestion; allowing thirty minutes for complete absorption, elapsed time periods were zero, fifteen, thirty, and sixty minutes. Thirty-five male university subjects were exposed to the control, small, and moderate dose, while an experimental subgroup of nine also took the criterion test following the large dose. The standardized work load consisted of intermittent maximal contractions of the forearm flexors at the rate of thirty per minute for six minutes. Parameters studied included initial strength, maximal strength, steady state or final strength, total work, fatigable work, and the mathematical rate of fatigue. The results of the statistical analysis revealed no significant main or interaction effects, and Williams concluded that the alcohol doses utilized in his study had no effect upon the strength or endurance variables under investigation.

In summary, the general results of contemporary research indicate that the acute ingestion of alcohol has little or no effect on subsequent tests of local muscular strength or endurance.

Effect on General Endurance

The research regarding the effect of alcohol upon general endurance capacity is more limited. In one of the earliest studies, Asmussen and Boje (26) investigated the influence of alcohol on the ability to perform maximal muscular work and concluded the effect was not significant. Two tasks on the bicycle ergometer were utilized, simulating a 100 meter dash and a 1500 meter run. They found that alcohol in small doses (25 g pure ethanol) had no effect, and alcohol in larger doses (75 g pure ethanol) had only a diminishing effect on the ability to perform maximal muscular work. Two other independent Scandinavian investigations (200, 214) also noted that small or moderate doses of alcohol did not affect physical working capacity. Although Nelson (377) noted a decrease in performance on seven gross motor tests following the intake of two and three ounces of pure ethanol, bicycle ergometer work time was one of the tests to show least change in efficiency when compared with control. Highly coordinated skills seemed to decrease most.

In a more recent investigation, Williams (547) studied the effect of a moderate dose (0.4 ml/lb) of pure ethanol upon time to exhaustion on a progressive bicycle ergometer work task. Ten conditioned male subjects underwent four test trials, two with a control dose and two with alcohol. He concluded that a moderate dose of alcohol neither adversely nor beneficially affected maximal endurance performance.

The results of these studies suggest that alcohol would not be a very effective ergogenic aid in athletic events characterized by all-out general muscular endurance.

In tests duplicating actual athletic events, both Hebbelinck (240) and Nelson (377) reported detrimental effects of alcohol upon speed. Hebbelinck found that a small dose decreased speed in the eighty meter dash almost 10 percent. No details were reported concerning the actual conduct of the test, but the difference may have been due to reaction time changes at the start. Aside from these two reports, no other literature was uncovered which directly studied the effect of alcohol on field tests of athletic performance.

When interpreting the results of experimentation involving the acute effects of alcohol on human performance, such as in single or double dose administration studies, one must be cautious not to generalize the findings to include the effect of chronic ingestion on performance. In experimentation regarding the acute effects, it appears that the possible limiting physiological manifestations mediated by alcohol during rest are abrogated during an exercise situation. However, the chronic ingestion of alcohol may produce certain physiological changes resulting in decreased endurance capacity. Since the liver is the main site for resynthesis of glycogen from lactic acid during exercise, the damaging effect chronic alcohol ingestion elicits in the liver may limit this process and thus allow higher blood lactate levels to accumulate during exercise. Lactic acid has been associated with the development of fatigue and consequently this result may hinder performance capacity. Burch (76) has indicated the chronic ingestion of ethanol exerts deteriorative effects on the mitochondria and other components of the heart, thus possibly hampering the oxygen consumption capacity of the myocardium, with a potential decrease in maximal cardiac output. deVries (134) indicated that the cardiac output is usually the limiting factor in determining the level at which work output can be maintained. Thus, the effects of chronic alcohol ingestion on human performance may be quite different than the results of testing which follow acute ingestion.

CHAPTER 4

DRUGS AFFECTING THE MUSCULAR SYSTEM

ANABOLIC STEROIDS

IT IS A WELL-KNOWN fact that the young male undergoes tremendous changes in body size and secondary sex characteristics at puberty. These changes are elicited by increased secretions of the male sex hormones, also known synonymously as androgenic hormones. All androgens are steroids and can be synthesized from cholesterol or acetyl coenzyme A. At least five different androgens are secreted by the adrenal gland and 4-androstene-3, 17,-dione is derived from the testes, but testosterone is secreted in such quantities that it is regarded as the primary androgen responsible for the male sex characteristics. Although testosterone exerts a number of physiological influences throughout the body, one of its primary effects is to increase protein synthesis, primarily in the skeletal muscles. Thus, testosterone may be utilized to increase body weight, and has been useful in certain diseases characterized by muscle wasting. This muscle building action of testosterone reflects its anabolic properties; however, testosterone also has potent androgenic properties, and if used therapeutically in women or children could lead to increased virilization. Therefore, biochemists have developed a number of synthetic compounds which maximize the anabolic properties of testosterone and minimize the androgenic effects.

In order to reduce the androgenic aspect of testosterone, its chemical configuration has been altered. The addition of a methyl group at position 4 generally favors increased anabolic activity and decreased androgenic activity. The increased anabolic activity leads to increased nitrogen retention in skeletal muscles and facilitates building of muscle tissue. However, the effectiveness of the anabolic steroid is dependent upon an adequate intake of calories and protein (188) as well as physical activity (19).

According to Vida (527), there is no truly 100 percent anabolic steroid yet; all have some androgenic properties. The relative proportion of each in any compound is determined by research with animals; the compound is usually compared to a standard such as testosterone, and its effectiveness is expressed as an anabolic-androgenic ratio. The following list contains some common compounds with proprietary names which are primarily anabolic in nature:

methandienone—(Dianabol®) (Danabol®)
ethyloestrenol—(Maxibolin®) (Orabolin®)
methandriol—(Stenediol®)
oxymesterone—(Oranabol®)
norethandrolone—(Nilevar®)
nandrolone phenpropionate—(Durabolin®)
nandrolone decanoate—(deca-Durabolin) (Abolon®)
oxandrolone—(Anavar®)
oxymetholone—(Adroyd®) (Anapolon®)
stanozolol—(Winstrol®) (Stromba®)

An excellent discussion regarding the structure, metabolic effects, activity theories, and therapeutic actions of the anabolic steroids may be found in *Androgens and Anabolic Agents* (527). Chapter 4 in particular covers the anabolic-androgenic ratio of most common anabolic steroids in use by 1967, while Chapter 5 lists over 600 androgenic and anabolic agents.

Use in Athletics

Anabolic steriods have found useful medical application in a variety of conditions, including certain anemias, osteoporosis, debilitating illnesses with muscle wasting, and growth defects. But nearly thirty-five years ago, Boje (56) contended the admin istration of sex hormones or preparations of the adrenal cortex could theoretically increase athletic performance. However, with the available evidence at that time, he was unable to make any sound conclusions. Within the past fifteen years, they have found broad application in the field of athletics. Recently, Cobley (102) indicated wide spread use of anabolic steroids among men involved in field events while Cooper (108) reported hearsay evidence that 80 percent of weight men use them.

The primary rationale for their use in athletic training would appear to be simple. The steroids can increase muscle mass, and since strength and muscle mass are proportional to a degree, strength will also increase; gains in power are usually associated with gains in strength. Therefore, in any athletic event where strength, power, or body mass are important, the use of anabolic steroids as an adjunct during training would seem to be effective. Several reports (369, 459) have indicated that these compounds may be more effectively applied to female athletes since women probably have greater percentual potential for strength development. On the other hand, the use of steroids during athletic training would be contraindicated in those sports where increased body weight is a disadvantage.

There is some disagreement as to the validity of this rationale. Freed and his colleagues (183) indicated self-administration of anabolic steroids by international level athletes is a common practice, and that the efficacy in improving performance is beyond doubt; this viewpoint has also been stated elsewhere (17). On the contrary, Shephard (466) stated that the rationale for administering anabolic steroids to mature young men is obscure, and there exists no objective evidence that performance is improved following their use. He contends that the muscle fibers of the well-trained athlete have already reached maximal diameter compatible with continued oxidation.

Nevertheless, the prevalence of these drugs in training programs for certain events has fostered legislation or statements against their use for athletic purposes by the Committee on Sports Medicine of the American Academy of Science, the Committee on the Medical Aspects of Sports of the American Medical

Association, the National Collegiate Athletic Association, the International Olympic Committee, the International Amateur Athletic Federation, the Food and Drug Administration, and even leading pharmaceutical firms (116).

One of the major problems facing the athletic governing bodies is detection of use. The athlete does not use anabolic steroids in conjunction with competition as amphetamines might be used, but rather during his training program. Consequently, he or she may cease using them prior to the actual event. However, a note (17) was made in 1971 that methods are being developed to detect the presence of steroids in the blood long after their administration has stopped. This would be an effective deterrent, but this author has not uncovered any evidence indicating the methods are currently available. Moreover, Frenkl and his associates (184) indicated that athletes eliminate steroids faster than untrained individuals. If steroid levels are to be determined by use of chromatography, they contend allowances must be made for the faster elimination rates in sportsmen.

Although the decision to legislate against steroid use in athletics was probably based upon matters of sports ethics, consideration was probably also given to the undetermined health hazards of prolonged steroid use by normal young men. Pharmacology texts have indicated that steroid abuse could stop growth, decrease testicular size and induce precocious puberty in prepubertal boys. Decreased testosterone production, reduction of testicular size and decreased libido could occur in pubertal males. Certain anabolic steroids, particularly those with an alkyl or alkynyl group in the alpha configuration at position 17, could cause liver damage of the cholestatic type. In a double-blind cross over study, Freed and his colleagues (183) noted that low (10 mg/day) and high (25 mg/day) dosages of Dianabol in comparison with a placebo caused several individual problems with blood pressure, prostatism and acne in ten weightlifters. Although their data were insufficient for statistical analysis, they concluded it would not be prudent to state that steroids at low levels have no adverse effects.

Needless to say, any athlete who uses anabolic steroids as an adjunct to his training program should do so only under the advice and supervision of a physician. Liver function tests should be conducted periodically.

Effect on Physical Performance

Literally thousands of studies have been conducted relative to the various pharmacological effects of androgenic and anabolic steroids. The following review contains those investigations with human and other animals that have implications for athletic performance. Reference is made to effects upon body weight and composition, strength, and other tests of physical working capacity.

Body Weight and Composition

It is an established fact that anabolic steroids are helpful in building muscle tissue, particularly in patients who are in need of such drug therapy. The steroids cause increased retention of nitrogen, a basic constituent of protein. Guyton (221) noted that testosterone injection increases the RNA concentration within the prostatic cell, which is soon followed by progressive increases in cellular protein. Several days later, the DNA concentration also increases. He speculated that the action of the hormone may be on the DNA in the nucleus. A similar mode of action probably exists in the skeletal musculature, thus increasing body weight. In addition, testosterone and the other anabolic steroids effectively help to reabsorb sodium and water from the distal renal tubules, thus increasing fluid retention. Because of the fluid retention, gains in body weight may not accurately reflect gains in skeletal musculature; therefore, body composition analyses are more appropriate.

The main question is not whether anabolic steroids can help to build muscle tissue, but rather can they augment the effects of exercise, since exercise in itself is anabolic in nature.

The results of several animal studies indicate that anabolic steroids do not, either alone or in combination with exercise, augment the muscular hypertrophy or body weight gains evinced by exercise alone. Wydra (553) studied the effect of Dianabol upon the skeletal musculature of mice. He assigned 139 mice to one of four groups: exercise, exercise plus Dianabol, Dianabol and control. The exercise involved running, and the study was conducted over a thirty-day period. The animals were then sacrificed and the triceps brachii was histologically examined in all the mice, and the quadriceps femoris in forty-nine mice. The results showed that both muscular training alone and the anabolic treatment alone produced musculature hypertrophy, with the exercise resulting in a lesser development. The exercise-anabolic group did not have significantly greater hypertrophy than the anabolic group. Palecek (392) reported no significant effect of dimethylandrostan upon the muscle weight of the normal rat gastrocnemius. Dosage was 5 mg/kg daily, but no indication of the length of training or exercise regimen was noted.

Murphy and Eagan (363) investigated the effect of anabolic steroids upon muscle size in lightly and heavily exercised rats. Twenty obese rats were trained in treadmill running for two weeks and then randomly assigned to four groups: Control and steroid groups were run 0.9 km/week to maintain treadmill familiarity whereas exercise and exercise steroid groups were run 9 km/week. Steroid and exercise steroid groups were given daily 0.3 mg each of stanozolol and methandrostenolone, and weekly 2.5 mg of nandrolone; all groups were given Purina Chow® ad libitum. At the end of the four week experiment, the control group had the greatest body weight, followed in order by the steroid, exercise, and exercise-steroid groups.

Brown and Pilch (68) randomly assigned eighteen rats (two each) to one of nine conditions involving the interaction of Dianabol and exercise. Drug levels were placebo, ½ mg/kg and 5 mg/kg; exercise levels were sedentary, high jumping and treadmill running. The experiment lasted six weeks. Although the analysis would be clouded by the small number of subjects in each treatment cell, the low dosage was the only condition that increased the weight of the levator ani, a muscle commonly evaluated in steroid investigations to determine anabolic effects. Feldscher (160) randomly assigned thirty-five Wistar rats to two groups and trained them five days/week for six weeks.

Training consisted of swimming a series of one-minute repetitions with thirty seconds rest between repetitions. In addition to the exercise, the experimental group received 10 mg/kg daily of oxandrolone. The results indicated no significant differences between the groups in either body weight, specific gravity or per cent body fat.

In these animal studies, one of the complicating factors is the nature of the exercise. Running and swimming are the methods most commonly used to exercise animals; muscular stress is moderate and prolonged, and in the process, calories are expended which would tend to reduce body weight and possibly negate the action of the steroids. Humans who desire to gain body weight utilize weight training techniques, exercises which place great stress on individual muscle groups and yet have low caloric expenditure. Thus, the insignificant effect of anabolic steroids on body weight in exercising animals may be due to the nature of the exercise.

One of the earliest studies concerning the combined effect of exercise and anabolic steroids on humans was conducted by Fowler and his associates in 1965 (178). In a well-designed study, they reported that Nibal®, a steroid, did not augment the effect of exercise upon various anthropometrical measurements. However, there were two major deficiencies in the study. First, the exercise described by the authors consisted of general physical conditioning; there was no indication as to the nature of the exercise, i.e. was it aerobic training or weight training. Secondly, no protein or caloric supplements were given to the subjects. In 1965, Saarne and others (444), following a series of experiments conducted under strictly controlled conditions, concluded that without an adequate supply of protein and calories, anabolic steroids will not produce a nitrogen retention effect. The extent of protein and caloric supply is of fundamental importance for the degree of nitrogen retention.

O'Shea (384) contends that the day of the Olympic athlete who is involved in strength events, and who competes with a minimum of weight training and a normal diet, is a phenomenon of the past. In order to effectively increase muscle mass for athletic purposes by the use of anabolic steroids, two other conditions are necessary; the athlete must be involved in a progressive resistive weight training program (PRE) and he must receive caloric and high quality protein supplements. The following studies are reviewed in light of these conditions.

Using a 2 x 2 factorial design involving no exercise and PRE as one variable and 6 mg stanozolol daily and placebo as the other variable, Casner and others (88) found that the steroids significantly increased the body weight in contrast to the placebo conditions. However, the lack of a significant change in specific gravity led to the conclusion that the greater body weight for the steroid group was probably due to a combined protein mass and water retention since the anabolic groups had a gain in total body water while the placebo group had a loss. No food supplements were administered. Fahey and Brown (157) evaluated the effect of nandrolone decanoate and weight training upon body composition. During the ten week study, 1.0 mg/kg nandrolone decanoate was injected intramuscularly at weeks two, five, and eight into the experimental subjects while the others received a sterile saline solution; both groups were involved in PRE training. No significant differences in body weight were noted, although the lean body mass increased equally in both groups. In this study, the dosage and method of administration of the steroid, as well as the absence of protein supplementation may have contributed to the insignificant gains.

In those studies which utilized PRE and protein supplementation, anabolic steroids augmented the effects of exercise upon body weight and muscular hypertrophy. Using twelve paired subjects, Johnson and O'Shea (275) reported that subjects receiving 10 mg/day of Dianabol in conjunction with 30 g of 92 percent protein/day attained significantly greater muscular hypertrophy and body weight than did subjects receiving only the protein; both groups trained by PRE for six weeks, and the drug treatment was administered during the last three weeks of training. No significant differences in adipose tissue were noted. A limitation to the study was the fact that it was not double-blind; the subjects knew they were receiving steroids. In a subsequent double-blind study, O'Shea (384) reported significantly greater body weight gains due to 10 mg/day methandrostenolone in comparison to a placebo group. Again, both groups received protein supplementation and undertook intensive PRE training. Using similar procedures, Johnson and others (276) reported a significant effect of 5 mg/day Dianabol upon body weight and several body circumferential measurements when compared to both a placebo and control group. Bowers and Reardon (63) also found that 10 mg/day Dianabol was significantly better than placebo treatment in regard to increased body weight and muscular girth.

Thus, the combination of progressive resistive weight training, caloric and protein supplementation, and anabolic steroids appears to effectively increase body mass. However, unless body mass in itself is an important consideration in athletic success, e.g. an interior lineman in football, the gain in musculature is useless unless there are concomitant gains in strength and power. Consequently, most of the studies already discussed have also analyzed the effects of anabolic steroids on strength, power, endurance, and other measures of physical working capacity. These results are covered in the following section.

Strength and Physical Working Capacity

The results of animal studies indicate that anabolic steroids exert no influence upon endurance capacity. In an early study, Maglio and others (337) noted that the intraperitoneal injection of 25 mg/kg of steranabol in trained adult guinea pigs caused an increase in the animals resistance to fatigue while running on a treadmill. In a more recent report, Murphy and Eagan (363) found that an exercise group and an exercise-steroid group of rats were equal in endurance capacity following a four week training period consisting of a 9 km/week run on a treadmill; the steroid group received 0.3 mg daily of both stanozolol and methandrostenolone and 2.5 mg weekly of nandrolone. Brown and Pilch (68) reported no significant effect of a small or large dose of Dianabol upon the jumping or treadmill running performance of mice trained over a six-week period. Feldscher (160), using a weighted swim to exhaustion test as the criterion measure of endurance, found no significant augmenting effect of 10 mg/kg oxandrolone above that elicited by exercise alone.

In humans, Guyton (221) indicated that testosterone has been described as a youth hormone, and may be effective in increasing strength levels of older men. In several older studies, the effect of testosterone on strength was investigated. Simonson and others (473) reported significant gains in dynamic and static work, finger ergography performance, and to a lesser degree, muscular strength, in four subjects following the administration of 25 mg methyltestosterone four times daily. However, it should be noted that the subjects were two castrates and two eunuchoids, who would probably benefit more than normal subjects from exogenous testosterone. In addition, a training effect may have confounded their results. In 1942, Samuels and his associates (446), using a replicated crossover study with four subjects, found that the administration of 50 mg methyltestosterone daily had no effect on grip strength; the drug was given over a four week period.

Using older subjects (48-67 years), Simonson and others (474) investigated the effect of 40 mg methyltestosterone administered daily upon strength and endurance. Although the experimental procedure was inadequate in terms of conventional methodology, the results did indicate a general tendency towards increased strength and endurance capacity due to the methyltestosterone. Hettinger (246) also reported significant increases in strength and physical working capacity of older subjects (65-70 years) following testosterone injections.

In more recent research, utilizing synthetic anabolic steroids rather than testosterone or methyltestosterone, the results suggest that steroids may be a useful adjunct to weight training for the development of strength. Again, caloric and protein supplementation appear to be necessary during the training program.

In a study involving muscular dystrophy patients, Fowler and his coworkers (179) reported that 0.25 mg androstenolone daily for one year had no therapeutic usefulness in improvement of muscular strength or physical working capacity. However, it is doubtful that these results may be extrapolated to normal subjects. In another study with ten college athletes and thirty-seven untrained college students, Fowler (178) revealed no significant effect of Nibal, an anabolic steroid, upon strength or physical working capacity. The subjects were assigned to one of four groups: placebo, steroid, placebo and exercise, and steroid and exercise. The study was double-blind and lasted sixteen weeks; exercise consisted of general physical conditioning five days/week for thirty minutes. Casner and others (88) used a similar four-group design with PRE three times weekly as the exercise variable and 6 mg stanozolol daily as the drug variable. In this double-blind study, the drug was administered on days 1 to 21 and 28 to 49 of the 56 day experimental period. The Elgin multiple angle testing machine was utilized to measure isometric strength in major muscle groups; tests were conducted on days 1, 28, and 56. No significant augmenting effect of the steroid was found. Fahey and Brown (157) reported no significant influence of deca-Durabolin upon either dynamic or isokinetic strength. Twenty-eight subjects were assigned to two groups, both undertaking a ten week PRE training program. The steroid group received 1.0 mg deca-Durabolin/kg at weeks 2, 5, and 8; the placebo group received sterile saline. Dosages were injected intramuscularly.

In the studies above, the absence of protein supplementation, low intensity of exercise programs and method of administration of the steroid may have been limiting factors.

Weiss and Muller (535) compared the effectiveness of 10 mg Dianabol daily for three weeks with a placebo upon dynamometer strength. They concluded that although there was no statistically significant difference between the two groups, individual changes indicated a connection between the use of anabolic steroids and strength gains. They also suggested the effect may be due to the interactions of drug dosage, protein supplementation and degree of training.

Using a replicated group design, O'Shea (383) indicated that the use of anabolic steroids alone as an ergogenic aid is ineffective in improving strength. One group received 10 mg methandrostenolone daily for three weeks while the other group received a placebo; treatments were reversed during the second three weeks of the study. No significant differences were noted on isometric strength as tested on a cable tensiometer. In three subsequent reports, O'Shea reported significant strength increases when steroids were used with PRE training and high quality protein supplements. Using only three weightlifters, O'Shea and Winkler (385) found that 10 mg oxandrolone daily increased static strength. The drug was administered during the first six weeks of an eleven week study, along with protein supplementation on the order of ½ g/kg/day. However, there was no placebo or control group used. In a more controlled study, Johnson and O'Shea (275) matched twelve subjects and exposed them to identical PRE training programs and supplementation of 30 g of 92 percent protein/day. The steroid group received 10 mg Dianabol/day. The results showed significantly greater dynamic and static strength levels for the steroid treatment group. Employing a double-blind placebo design, O'Shea (384) studied the effects of four weeks of anabolic steroid treatment on strength levels of experienced weightlifters. Twenty subjects were used, paired according to strength levels, and assigned randomly to the treatment (10 mg/day methandrostenolone) or placebo groups. All subjects undertook identical PRE training programs in conjunction with protein supplementation. The criterion test was a one-repetition maximum on the bench press and squat lifts. The results indicated the steroid group was significantly stronger in both strength tests as well as body weight gains. It may be conceivable that the steroid group, if they were cognizant of their individual body weight gains, might have experienced a psychological effect, so important in all-out strength tests.

In a well-controlled double-blind placebo experiment, Johnson and his coworkers (276) pre-trained twenty-four subjects and then randomly assigned them to a treatment (5 mg Dianabol/day) or placebo group; seven other subjects served as a control group. All subjects continued to train by PRE methods, while the treatment and placebo groups also consumed 20 g of 92 percent protein powder daily. The steroid group had significantly greater dynamic and static strength gains in comparison to the control and placebo groups. Bowers and Reardon (63) studied the effects of 10 mg Dianabol upon the strength development of eighteen experienced weightlifters. Subjects were matched according to age, size, and strength and assigned to the treatment or placebo group. Following a pre-test the subjects engaged in a six-week PRE training program. All subjects received 30 g of 90 percent protein supplement daily. The placebo and Dianabol were given during the last twenty-one days of training. The steroid group experienced significantly greater gains in bench press and squat tests than did the placebo group.

Ariel (20) investigated the effect of Dianabol upon skeletal muscle contractile force by testing maximal weight lifting. Six varsity weightlifters were studied over a four month period. During the first several weeks, subjects trained with specific lifts and executed maximums each week. From the eighth to eleventh weeks all subjects received placebo pills, but were told they contained 10 mg Dianabol. During weeks 12 to 15 a double-blind procedure was used; three subjects continued to receive the placebos, while the other three received 10 mg Dianabol. Ariel analyzed the data by comparing the slopes of the regression line for the three periods of the study: training, placebo, and steroid periods. His results indicated the steroid group was able to exert a greater maximal contractile force in the steroid period when compared to the placebo period. Also, the rate of progress for the steroid group was higher during the steroid period as compared to the placebo group, which did not significantly alter their rate of progress during the last eight weeks of the study. In the same study, Ariel also investigated the effects of the steroid upon reflex components; the results are reported elsewhere (22). He noted that anabolic steroids significantly decreased the reflex time, primarily by its action on the motor component as contrasted to the latency period. Thus, the steroid appeared to facilitate the time period between the recording of the muscle action potential and subsequent mechanical movement. Although it appears out of context here in the discussion of strength, it was included as an aside since it was a part of his study on strength and was the only study of this nature reported in the literature.

Imhof (265), summarizing several German studies, indicated that the administration of anabolic steroids to athletes, in conjunction with suitable training and an appropriate diet, can produce an additional increase in strength by incorporating protein into the skeletal muscle.

Ariel (21) investigated the retention effect of anabolic steroids upon dynamic strength as measured by the one repetition-maximum technique. Twenty male weightlifters were trained for eight weeks, one group receiving methandrostenolone and the other training without the drug. A fifteen week detraining period followed the training period. Although both groups significantly increased their strength during the training period, only the control group experienced a significant decrease in strength after detraining; the steroid group maintained their strength levels. The results of this study may have implications for detection techniques; in order to effectively detect the prior use of steroids in athletes, they will have to account for this retention effect. In other words, can steroids be detected six weeks after discontinuation?

Richardson and Bassett (422), in a rather unique experiment, trained African green monkeys to exert force and raise a weight on a pulley apparatus. Following a thirty day training period, they initiated an experiment with three monkeys who had established consistent base line strength levels. Using a counterbalanced design, each animal was subjected to three treatment conditions: placebo, anabolic steroid (Dianabol), and a nonsteroid weight gaining drug (Periactin®). Thus, each animal served as his own control. The drug dosages were the equivalent of 20 mg/daily Dianabol for humans, considered to be a heavy dose. All animals trained three months on each treatment condition; high protein supplements were administered daily. Since the animals were doing strength training, strength naturally increased. However, the general results indicated that the anabolic steroids elicited greater strength gains than the control, but Periactin, to the surprise of the investigators, was more effective than steroids in the development of strength. Moreover, when the animals ceased taking the drug, the return of strength to baseline values was rapid under steroid treatment, but Periactin was effective in maintaining attained strength levels.

Biopsy analyses are being conducted in an attempt to ascertain the underlying mechanisms.

In several of the aforementioned studies, the effect of anabolic steroids upon physical working capacity or maximal oxygen uptake was also investigated. Without alluding to the details of these studies, the results will be indicated. The interested reader may refer back to the prior paragraphs for information on drug dosage and methodology. Johnson and O'Shea (275) reported an unexpected increase in max VO_2 in the steroid group. They used the Astrand oxygen uptake test, but the reported mean values for the workload were less than 1050 kpm, which are relatively small values to elicit max VO_2 in trained men. Apparently they used the predictive test, which has wide variability. In a subsequent report (383) no significant effect of steroids were noted on max VO_2 as estimated by the Astrand-Rhyming test. Bowers and Reardon (63), Johnson and others (276), and Fahey and Brown (157) all reported no significant effect of anabolic steroids upon max VO_2. On the other hand, Albrecht and Albrecht (10) reported that the daily administration of anabolic steroids appeared to have a beneficial effect on PWC_{170} in comparison to a control group. The PWC_{170} test was conducted on subjects at increasing altitudes (sea level, 4300 m and 6200 m). Although the PWC_{170} decreased during ascent, the group receiving the anabolic steroid scored significantly better than a placebo or vitamin group. However, the PWC_{170} test is submaximal and does not offer an accurate measure of max VO_2.

Only two studies were uncovered that investigated the effect of steroids upon a simulated athletic event. O'Shea (383) and O'Shea and Winkler (385) reported no effects of anabolic steroids, in conjunction with training for swimming, upon the swimming speed or endurance of competitive swimmers. The details of experimental methodology may be found in preceding paragraphs.

In summary, it would appear that anabolic steroids may be an effective adjunct to weight training and protein supplementation for sports that involve increased muscle mass, strength, and power. Although the evidence is not entirely conclusive, the available research does indicate increased strength levels if steroids are taken in conjunction with a proper training and dietary regimen. Needless to say, the athlete should take the drugs only under a physician's guidance and in accordance with rules and regulations pertaining to their use by the appropriate athletic governing body.

ASPARTATES

Use in Athletics

Potassium (K) and magnesium (Mg) aspartate are salts of asparaginic acid, a dibasic nonessential amino acid. Consequently, they are probably better classified as a food than as a drug, but are included in this discussion because they have been ascribed pharmacological actions to help prevent fatigue. They have been used therapeutically to relieve the general fatigue syndrome, fatigue resulting from long marches, and even in the labor fatigue associated with birth (555). Fujioka and his colleagues (189) indicated that aspartates could have wide application to sports as a routine means to counteract fatigue.

Although aspartates have been utilized to counteract the fatigue developing from physical work, their mode of action is still unclear. They are included in this chapter based on the glycogen enhancement rationale described by Ahlborg, but could just as readily be placed in the following chapter if the blood ammonia theory was chosen.

Golding (209) and Cutinelli (125) indicated that the theoretical benefit from aspartic acid salts may be due to their effect of reducing blood ammonia levels, which might be involved in the etiology of fatigue. Ahlborg (8) suggested that aspartates may accelerate the resynthesis of ATP, phosphocreatine, and glycogen in the muscle, and may also exert a glycogen sparing effect; these factors may enhance endurance capacity. It should be noted that although blood ammonia levels do increase during physical activity, no definite cause and effect relationship has been proven relative to their effect upon the development of fatigue. On the other hand, substantial evidence (7, 27) has supported the concept that increased muscle glycogen content will prolong work time to exhaustion.

In either case, however, their usefulness in sports, if any, would primarily be in endurance events.

Effect on Physical Working Capacity

In 1963, the Council on Drugs of the American Medical Association (114) indicated that although several reports have engendered the idea that aspartic acid salts are useful in the management of fatigue, no objective evidence is available to substantiate that claim. The additional limited research conducted within the past ten years would resubstantiate this statement, especially in relationship to exhausting fatigue as experienced in athletic endurance events.

Experiments with Animals

Laborit (314) conducted one of the original studies measuring the effects of aspartates upon work capacity. Using a double swim test to exhaustion, with 2½ hours rest between tests, aspartates apparently increased the exhaustion swim time in the experimental group of rats. In addition, blood ammonia levels were higher in the control rats as compared to the aspartate group; this finding may have given rise to the blood ammonia theory discussed above. Rosen and his associates (437) reported similar findings. They tested the effects of 10 g K and Mg aspartates/kg upon swim time to exhaustion. Ten rats were randomly assigned to the experimental and control groups. Using eight similar trials, or a total of 36 control and 36 aspartate rats (eight rats were eliminated), the results showed a 15 percent advantage in swim time to exhaustion in the aspartic group. After graphically plotting the data, the authors believed the aspartates were primarily beneficial to rats who initially had lesser endurance capacity rather than those who had strong endurance capacity at the beginning. It should also be noted that the data from eight animals were discarded, a fact that may have altered the significant results.

Barnes and others (36) also reported prolongation of the swim to exhaustion time in rats following the administration of aspartates. However, they did note that complicating factors such as age, diet, water temperature, and weighted tails, although carefully controlled, may have produced a variability between groups and thus led to the significant results.

Matoush and his colleagues (349) studied the effects of aspartates on physical performance during five separate experiments. The first test involved a simple swim to exhaustion of forty rats, twenty control and twenty receiving 500 mg aspartates; the water temperature was 17° C. Experiment two was exactly the same, only the water temperature was 25° C. The third experiment involved four dogs in the swim test, the experimental animals receiving 1.0 g aspartates. Experiments four and five utilized aspartate therapy; forty rats were assigned to either a placebo or aspartate (500 mg/daily) group. The aspartates were administered five days/week for six weeks. Experiment four consisted of a swim to exhaustion, while experiment five involved a double swim to exhaustion. Analyses in all five swim experiments revealed no significant differences between the aspartates and control or placebo conditions.

Experiments with Humans

Three separate medical reports indicated that aspartates were effective in alleviating the general symptoms of fatigue. Shaw and others (463), using a double-blind placebo design with 163 subjects, reported subjective and objective evidence as to the efficacy of aspartic acid salts in the relief of fatigue in patients. Kruse (313) reported similar findings, although noting several methodological problems which might influence his conclusion. Kondo (305) also noted beneficial subjective sensations following aspartate therapy. However, these three reports involved sedentary subjects experiencing general fatigue, and the results cannot be readily applied to intense physical activity.

Several reports have indicated an ergogenic effect of aspartates on human physical work capacity. Fujioka and others (190) indicated that the degree of physiological fatigue encountered in a thirty kilometer full-pack march was decreased due to the ingestion of aspartic acid salts. Fukui and others (191) suggested K and Mg aspartates were effective in the recovery from muscular fatigue, but the design of these studies with only an N=3 and questionable methods for objectively determining muscular fatigue renders their conclusions doubtful. Vial (526) reported aspartates are effective in counteracting neuromuscular fatigue in athletes by facilitating recovery following effort. However, Fallis and others (158) noted his research was rather uncontrolled. Using field tests, Fujioka and others (189) studied the effects of aspartates on the performance of military personnel in the 500 meter run, 1000 meter run, marathon running, and Ranger training. They noted that the accumulation of fatigue, particularly that which leads to a state of exhaustion, was prevented by the administration of the aspartate preparation. However, it was not revealed whether the actual time performance or the various running events were significantly improved by aspartates.

In more controlled laboratory research, the general results indicate aspartates will not benefit the trained subject who is motivated for work. Ahlborg and his coworkers (8), using six subjects with average physical fitness levels for Sweden, studied the influence of aspartates on the capacity for prolonged standardized physical exercise. The subjects were tested four times on a bicycle ergometer workload that was designed to elicit exhaustion in about ninety minutes. A double-blind placebo design was used. Tablets were taken every sixth hour during the study. Placebo tablets were taken on days 1, 2, and 4; aspartates (1.75 g tablets) were consumed on day 3. The aspartates appeared to increase the capacity for prolonged exercise as the mean value for the aspartate was 128 minutes as compared to 93.7, 85.3, and 88.3 minutes for the three placebo days. The authors suggested the increase was due to the effect of aspartates upon the various sources of energy in the skeletal muscle, enhancing the resynthesis of ATP, creatine phosphate and glycogen. The increase due to aspartates was approximately 40 to 50 percent greater than on placebo days, a finding that is difficult to digest. It is conceivable that the nature of the workload, i.e. submaximal since the recorded heart rates were only 150 to 160, may have been subject to modification through psychological processes. If the subjective effects reported earlier were noted by these subjects, it may have influenced their performance. In addition, a counterbalanced design would have been more appropriate. Nevertheless, the design was good and the results are suggestive of an ergogenic effect of aspartic acid salts.

Nagle and his colleagues (371) tested the effects of aspartates on fatiguing running exercise. Four subjects, two trained and two untrained, undertook three work tests on a treadmill: rested, following a sixty-minute cross country run, and again following an additional forty minute run. The subjects were trained to the task and then placed upon a Spartase® regimen consisting of 2000 mg K and Mg aspartate daily for two weeks; one subject received the dosage for one week. The results indicated that the treatment had no effect on the trained subjects, but did appear to increase the performance capacity of the untrained men; these findings are similar to a previous study with animals (437). However, the authors did note that limitations, such as the small number of subjects and possible training effect, precluded any generalizations concerning the anti-fatigue effects of Spartase.

Using a treatment by subjects design, Evans and Caldwell (155) subjected five highly motivated subjects to a physical work test of strength and endurance involving the use of an arm dynamometer. Each subject undertook the test eight times, four with placebo and four following the administration of 2000 mg K and Mg aspartates/day for four days. A double-blind procedure was used. Although all subjects were able to identify the subjective effects of the aspartates, the analysis revealed no significant effect upon strength or muscular endurance. The authors indicated the aspartates were ineffective because highly motivated subjects were used. They also suggested the salts may be effective with low motivated groups, possibly because the conversion of aspartates to glutamic acid may have an effect on the CNS and increase motivational levels.

In a controlled study (inmates in the Maryland State Penitentary were subjects), Fallis and her colleagues (158) studied the effect of aspartates upon the performance of twenty-six experienced weight lifters. The subjects were athletically inclined and considered to be in peak condition. Half the subjects were given placebos for ten days while the other half received 1 g/daily of K and Mg aspartic salts. This procedure was reversed for a second ten-day period. On the tenth day of each treatment session, maximal endurance scores were obtained on squats, bench press, military press, and grip ergograph performance. The subject's subjective evaluation of his condition and perception of time needed for recovery were also noted. The results indicated no significant differences between the aspartate and placebo conditions for any of the parameters, except the subjective perception of their physical condition was higher under the placebo treatment; this would contradict previous findings relative to subjective feelings of enhancement following aspartates.

The results of the two previous studies may be due to the nature of the induced fatigue. Both studies appeared to have studied local muscular fatigue with a heavy resistance, whereas the hypothetical benefit from aspartates would be in more moderate prolonged aerobic tasks. However, their results do support the viewpoint that aspartates are not effective ergogenic aids.

Consolazio and others (107) studied the effects of aspartates (500 mg K and Mg salts twice daily) upon oxygen uptake, oxygen debt, and physical working capacity. Twelve men were randomly assigned to either a placebo or aspartate group and underwent two weeks of training, five weeks of aspartate therapy, and two weeks recovery. All subjects exercised thirty minutes daily at 4 mph with a 3.5 percent grade on a treadmill. Towards the end of the aspartate period, subjects were exposed to a maximal test on the treadmill (7.0 mph, 8.0% grade). The results indicated no significant differences in oxygen consumption, oxygen debt, or physical fitness levels. The authors concluded that aspartates are not beneficial to human endurance performance, at least as determined by their run to exhaustion test. However, no times to exhaustion were reported and it appears that the physical fitness level was determined by the Harvard scoring system, which apparently uses recovery pulse rates to assess fitness.

In summary, while aspartates may have some application for the relief of subjective fatigue, their use does not appear to elicit any significant increase in physical working capacity of trained subjects. However, as noted by both Golding (209) and deVries (134), more research, especially with highly trained athletes, is warranted since aspartates appear to produce no serious adverse side effects.

CHAPTER 5

DRUGS AFFECTING THE
CARDIOVASCULAR SYSTEM

S INCE THE CARDIOVASCULAR system is involved in athletic events characterized by general endurance, such as distance running, swimming or bicycling, numerous attempts have been made to increase its efficiency for athletic competition. The technique of blood doping, the utilization of alkaline salts, and the administration of certain cardiovascular drugs are discussed in light of their potential ergogenic effects on the cardiovascular system during exercise.

BLOOD DOPING

Use in Athletics

Endurance athletes usually have well-developed cardiovascular systems and are able to produce more energy over a prolonged period of time due to their high maximal oxygen uptake capacity (max VO_2). Shephard (465) indicated that max VO_2 is normally limited by physiological rather than biochemical processes, and concluded that overall conductance of oxygen can be augmented by an increase in blood hemoglobin concentrations and/or increased cardiac output.

The removal of 500 to 1000 ml blood, with concomitant loss of hemoglobin, has been shown to significantly reduce physical working capacity and max VO_2 (29, 149, 290, 439). On the other hand, although no definite conclusions have been made,

Balke and others (30, 31) suggested that athletic training at altitude may enhance endurance performance upon subsequent return to sea level due to increased blood volume, red blood cells and hemoglobin. It is an established fact that chronic endurance training and acclimatization to altitude will elicit, respectively, increased blood volume and red blood cell volume (30, 255, 445, 477). Oscai and others (382) suggested that increases in maximal oxygen uptake through training are associated with increases in total blood volume. Thus, an increased blood volume may contribute to increased performance levels in prolonged aerobic activity.

A recent report in *Track and Field News* (53) noted that the technique of blood doping may already be in use by international athletes in attempts to increase endurance capacity. In essence, blood doping is the infusion of blood into an athlete. It may be his own blood, which has been withdrawn three weeks prior, or other cross-matched blood. Either whole blood or packed RBC's may be injected; the volume used would depend on the weight of the subject. The report was based upon recent research by Bjorn Ekblom and his associates.

Ekblom (53) indicated blood doping is not against any rules and probably never could be, probably due to the difficulty in detection. He had been offered 100,000 Swedish crowns for his exact method, and international track athletes expressed interest in the technique. However, Ekblom contended the aim of his research was not to find a perfect way to dope athletes, but to study the different parameters that will influence the oxygen transport system chain and the general physical performance capacity.

The theory underlying blood doping is relatively simple. By increasing either the blood volume and/or RBC and hemoglobin concentration, the athlete might possibly have greater oxygen carrying capacity. The physiological state could be advantageous in endurance events.

The technique may also have some therapeutic value, as deWijn and others (136) noted approximately 7 percent of the 1968 Netherland's Olympic team had some type of anemia.

A number of studies has been conducted relative to changes in resting heart rate, cardiac output and oxygen consumption following the infusion of whole blood or blood components, and several have investigated physiological modifications during exercise. Only a few studies have directly evaluated the usefulness of blood reinfusion as a possible ergogenic aid for athletes.

Physiological Effects of Blood Infusion

Plasma volume is integrally related to RBC volume; if the RBC volume is markedly reduced, the plasma compartment expands so that total blood volume remains relatively constant. Conversely, any attempt to increase blood volume forcibly by infusion of fluids, plasma, or cells is promptly countered by restoration of blood volume to previous levels (34). The infusion of 500 ml or more whole blood would produce a transient hypervolemia, expanding the blood volume in proportion to the individual's circulating blood. Since the exchange rate of fluid across the capillary wall is high, the reinjected plasma compartment, which is 91 percent water, would undergo rapid reduction. In hemorrhage, Berne and Levy (50) noted that reabsorption of tissue fluid into the vascular system may occur at the rate of .25 ml/minute/kg body weight, which approximates one liter of fluid per hour in a normal man (70 kg). If the reverse occurs during attempts at blood expansion, the original 500 ml blood volume would be reduced to approximately 250 ml of RBC; proportional decreases would occur in larger volumes of reinjected blood. Adjustments in cell volume are made more slowly over periods of days or weeks. Consequently, the resultant hematological state following the injection of either whole blood or packed red cells would be normovolemic polycythemia. Hemoglobin concentration in the average adult is raised about 1 g/100 ml blood by the transfer of 540 ml whole blood.

In 1922, Meck and Eyster (353) inferred that hypervolemia did not change cardiac output because there is no measurable increase in heart size. Moreover, they noted the plethora induced by blood transfusions was accommodated by the opening of capillaries and veins. However, more recent investigations have reported that the infusion of whole blood and other rheological compounds into dogs significantly increased the resting cardiac output. DeCristofaro and Liu (130) found that 20 to 22 ml whole blood/kg increased resting cardiac output, heart rate, and stroke volume in dogs. Ferguson and others (161) reported similar findings. Murray and others (366) also noted that systemic oxygen transport in ml/kg/minute was significantly higher in hypervolemic as contrasted to normovolemic dogs. Since the arterial oxygen saturation was not different under the two conditions, they attributed the increase to the greater cardiac ouput and decreased peripheral vascular resistance. Robinson and his associates (429) found that the infusion of 1000 to 1200 ml blood increased the cardiac output nearly 1500 ml/minute in six men.

Although hypervolemia might occur immediately after reinfusion, the competing athlete who received a blood infusion would probably compete in a state of normovolemic polycythemia, as the equivalent of the infused plasma volume would diffuse through the capillary walls. The increased RBC concentration would account for greater hemoglobin concentration and hence potential benefits for an exercise situation. On the other hand, normovolemic polycythemia during rest has been shown to elicit a decreased cardiac output, increased peripheral vascular resistance, increased blood viscosity, and decreased venous return (365, 421, 536). Replogle and Merrill (421) noted a reduced peripheral oxygen content, inferring that the increased oxygen carrying capacity of the blood due to hemoconcentration was not sufficient to counterbalance the effect of the reduced cardiac output. Guyton and Richardson (222) indicated that polycythemia reduced the minute RBC flow to the tissues due to decreased venous return. They concluded that oxygen transport was at a maximum, in dogs, at a hematocrit of 40, and elevating the hematocrit apparently was not beneficial. During rest, Weisse and his colleagues (536) also noted that normovolemic polycythemia decreased cardiac output and oxygen transport. Thus, the increased RBC concentration during rest appears to be detrimental to oxygen transport. Indeed, Replogle and Merrill

(421) indicated the rheological disadvantages of polycythemia at rest outweigh the advantages of an increased oxygen carrying capacity since acutely induced polycythemia appears to cause significant decreases in tissue perfusion and availability of oxygen to the tissues, enough to cause a shift in cellular metabolism towards anaerobic pathways.

During exercise the sympathetic nervous system mediates a variety of physiological adjustments in the cardiovascular system which may override the effects of blood infusion at rest. The onset and continuation of exericse produces an increased cardiac output through increases in both heart rate and stroke volume, increased arterial-venous oxygen difference, vasodilation in active muscles and vasoconstriction in the inactive musculature, adjustments in the regional distribution of blood, decreased blood volume, and increased hemoglobin concentration (27, 134, 503).

Weisse and his associates (536) studied the cardiovascular effects of normovolemic polycythemia during exercise. Using three dogs, the animals responded to exercise by quantitative changes similar to those during normocythemic exercise. Thus, although they noted decreased cardiac output and oxygen transport during rest with polycythemia, these values were normally not affected during exercise.

Williams and others (546), using twenty male athletes, concluded that the infusion of either 500 ml whole blood, 275 ml packed RBC's, or 225 ml plasma exerted no significant effect upon submaximal exercise heart rate, oxygen consumption or oxygen pulse.

In one of the most pertinent studies regarding physiological effects of blood doping during exercise, Robinson and his associates (429) studied the influence of acute blood volume expansion upon maximal cardiac output and maximal oxygen consumption. Six male subjects augmented their blood by 1000 to 1200 ml of their own blood. Although the central venous pressure was higher, the blood expansion had no effect upon either maximal cardiac output or oxygen uptake during treadmill exercise. They indicated that all of the infused blood is accommodated in the venous compartments, the capacitance vessels. The authors concluded that blood volume is not a factor which limits cardiac response to maximal exercise in normal subjects.

In addition, the oxygen carrying capacity of the blood has yet to be substantiated as a limiting factor in endurance capacity. True, decreases in hemoglobin concentration such as occur in anemia may restrict performance capability, but does the augmenting effect of blood reinfusion to the highly trained athlete confer any additional benefits? The tissues may be the limiting factor in aerobic performance and may only extract the amount of oxygen necessary to sustain a given metabolic level.

Effect on Physical Working Capacity

Five reports have been uncovered which investigated the effect of blood infusion on PWC. Three of the studies used submaximal exercise tests as the criterion measure for PWC, while the other two used maximal tests.

In 1947, Pace and others (390) induced a polycythemia in five normal men by the infusion of 2000 ml of 50 percent suspension of compatible erythrocytes at a rate of 500 ml/day for four days. The hematocrit value rose from 46.2 to 58.3 percent, and the polycythemia lasted fifty days. The oxygen carrying capacity of the arterial blood was increased 23 percent. Using the pulse rate during submaximal work as the criterion measure for adjustment to simulated hypoxic levels, the authors concluded that the transfusion conferred an advantage to the subjects when exposed to a simulated altitude.

Gullbring and his colleagues (220) used the PWC_{170}, a submaximal test, to investigate the withdrawal and reinfusion effect of approximately 10 percent of the blood volume in six physicians. Age range was 26 to 51. Performance was adversely affected on tests the day following withdrawal. The blood was reinfused seven days after withdrawal, and a marked improvement in PWC_{170} was noted one hour post-infusion. However, it appears retests were conducted each day following withdrawal, which may have elicited a training effect.

In a related study, Albrecht and Albrecht (10) reported that solcoseryl, a liquid antigen-free nonprotein extract from the blood of young calves, increased PWC_{170} scores during altitude ascent. Again, a training effect may have occurred due to the nature of their experimental design.

Ekblom and his associates (149) studied the effects of blood loss and subsequent reinfusion on the PWC of seven nonathletic subjects. Three subjects, group I, underwent a single venesection of 800 ml blood, while four subjects, group II, lost 1200 ml during three withdrawals of 400 ml each. Base line values for heart rate, oxygen uptake, submaximal and maximal work parameters were determined prior to the blood loss. PWC and max VO_2 decreased substantially following withdrawal. Approximately four weeks later the blood was reinfused. Subjects in group I were retested just prior to reinfusion. In this group, the increased blood volume caused a significant increase in max VO_2, hemoglobin and maximal work time. The same increase in max VO_2 was not noted in group II since no preinfusion data was available from the preceding day. However, they did experience substantial increases in maximal work time and hemoglobin when compared to base line values. Although it was a highly sophisticated study, the data may have been confounded by a training effect and lack of a control group; in addition, no indication of a double-blind design was noted.

Williams and his colleagues (549) evaluated the effects of reinjected hematological components on endurance capacity and maximal heart rate. Twenty male athletes, mostly distance runners, were pre-tested on a maximal treadmill run and assigned to one of four groups: whole blood (500 ml), packed RBC's (275 ml), plasma (225 ml), and control. Five hundred ml of blood was withdrawn from the subjects in the three experimental groups; the control group also went through the venipuncture protocol. All subjects were blindfolded during the withdrawal and reinfusion stages of the investigation; a double-blind design was utilized. Twenty-one days following withdrawal, the hematological components were infused into the appropriate groups. The maximal test was readministered approximately two hours post-infusion, two days post-infusion, and six days post-infusion. A two-way ANOVA revealed no significant effects due to treatments, and the authors concluded the infusion of whole blood, packed RBC's, or plasma, at least in the quantities utilized in their study, had no differential effect upon endurance capacity or maximal heart rate. It should be noted that they used only 500 ml of blood, which is almost one-half the value used by Ekblom in the previously cited report.

Although some may contend that the withdrawal and reinjection of an athlete's blood under controlled conditions may significantly increase endurance capability, the available literature does not appear to provide physiological rationale or sufficient objective evidence to substantiate that contention.

ALKALINE SALTS

Use in Athletics

One of the theoretical contributing factors in the development of fatigue during exercise is increased acidosis, primarily due to lactic acid production during anaerobic work. Lactic acid is the anaerobic end product of glycolysis, and it may be produced in substantial quantities in the muscle during high intensity exercise; the lactate level then rises in the blood stream. During heavy exercise, the lactic acid component accounts for the majority of the oxygen debt, and deVries (134) indicated that the magnitude of the oxygen debt which may be attained by an athlete may be a very important factor in heavy endurance work. He further noted that the size of the oxygen debt may be limited by the blood pH.

The blood pH is normally in the range of 7.35 to 7.45, but may decrease to 7.0 during exercise. The ingestion of alkaline salts, such as sodium citrate, sodium bicarbonate, or potassium citrate, has been shown to displace the pH upwards during a resting state. The theory behind their use, therefore, is relatively simple. If the lowered blood pH during exercise is a contributing causative factor in the etiology of fatigue, then the use of alkaline salts will increase the normal alkaline reserve of the blood and help buffer the acid produced during exercise. This may keep the pH high in the muscle tissue as well as the blood, thus maintaining a more homeostatic condition for the functioning of the enzymes involved in muscular contraction. Astrand and Rodahl (27) noted that the reduced alkaline reserve following acclimitization to altitude may be a factor behind decreases in anaerobic capacity; thus, it follows logically that an increased alkaline reserve may increase anaerobic capacity.

The primary alkaline salts which have been used as ergogenic aids are the citrates and bicarbonates of sodium and potassium. Upon oral ingestion they eventually elevate the blood pH. Other salts such as sodium phosphate and sodium sulfate would be effective, but they would have to be administered intravenously since they are not absorbed too well from the gastrointestinal tract. Organic compounds such as THAM (trometamol or trihydroxymethylaminomethane) have been used medically to treat metabolic and respiratory acidosis, and thus are similar in action to the alkalinizers. However, THAM is also diuretic, and could have an adverse effect on performance capacity by decreasing the blood volume.

Although the increased pH would appear to confer a physiological advantage during exercise, it may also be disadvantageous. The increased pH, due to its effect upon the oxygen dissociation curve, will decrease the ability of hemoglobin to release oxygen at the tissue level. However, the primary use of alkalinizers may be in those events characterized by high levels of anaerobic work, i.e. maximal effort for two minutes or less. Thus, the effect on the oxygen dissociation curve may not be important.

The theoretical physiological rationale for the use of alkaline salts in athletics appears to be logical, and aside from the possible development of flatulence, there appears to be no serious side effects associated with normal dosages. However, only a few reported studies have been uncovered.

Effect on Physical Working Capacity

In the earliest investigation, Dennig and others (132) indicated that a runner starting in a state of alkalosis, as compared to a normal state, may be able to accumulate a larger oxygen debt. However, they noted their work rate was not severe enough to test their hypothesis. Dill and his associates (137) reported that the ingestion of sodium bicarbonate did increase oxygen debt capability, noting an approximate 20 percent increase. Dennig (131) later reported significant increases in treadmill and bicycle ergometer endurance times of subjects ingesting alkaline salts according to a specified regimen. His refined dosages included 5.0 g sodium citrate, 3.5 g sodium bicarbonate, and 1.5 g potassium citrate taken after each meal for two days prior to the event; no dosage should be taken five hours prior to exercise. Dennig stressed the importance of this time schedule since the body may otherwise adjust to the salts. One of the limitations of this study was the fact that only moderately trained subjects were used.

Karpovich (291), although not divulging too many details, reported that Dennig's formula had no significant effect on performance of college swimmers.

In a field study, Johnson and Black (277) studied the effects of alkaline salts and glucose on the performance of champion high school cross country runners during a competitive season. The athletes, age range 16 to 19, ran the same 1.5 mile course eight times competitively during the season. They received either a placebo or experimental compound four hours prior to all meets except one; in the one exception, the dosage was administered 2.5 hours before competition. The rotation was such that each subject was tested twice with each of the following substances: (a) glucose, 2 ounces, (b) sodium citrate, 5 g, (c) sodium bicarbonate, 3.5 g, and potassium citrate, 1.5 g, and (d) sodium acid phosphate, 3 g, and glucose, 2.4 ounces. It should be noted that this procedure does not adhere to the regimen, either in dosages or time factors, advocated by Dennig. Subjects were unaware of the nature of the study and the criterion measure was time to run the course. The results indicated no significant effect due to the experimental drugs. However, Johnson and Black stated that the temperature range throughout the fall season (39°-91° F) may have influenced the results.

As indicated previously, alkalinizers may be more effective in work which is primarily anaerobic in nature, i.e. maximal work capacity in events of two minutes or less. Astrand and Rodahl (27) indicated a 50-50 percent derivation of energy from aerobic and anaerobic sources at maximal work for two minutes. The percentages become, respectively, 70-30 for maximal work of four minutes, and 90-10 for ten minutes. Thus, alkalinizers would appear to confer a physiological advantage primarily in events of short duration at maximal work rates. Examples would be the 800 meter or half-mile runs.

With this concept in mind, Margaria and his associates (342) recently studied the effect of 3.24 g sodium bicarbonate, sodium citrate and potassium citrate upon supramaximal exercise performance (10 MPH with 10% grade) of twelve normal men; there were four athletes, four active men, and four with no sports activity. Time to exhaustion was the criterion measure. The alkali salts had no significant effect upon performance. Blood lactic acid levels also were not affected. A few additional tests with massive doses of alkaline salts (12 g sodium bicarbonate) were conducted, and although endurance time increased up to 5.8 percent, this finding was not statistically significant. Therefore, the authors concluded that the alkaline salts had no appreciable influence on performance capacity of a supramaximal type.

In summary, the results indicate that alkaline salts are ineffective as ergogenic aids with trained athletes. However, more objective evidence is needed. Since these substances are relatively harmless, further research may be desirable.

CARDIOVASCULAR DRUGS

As cardiovascular disease has been one of the prime causes of death throughout the years, considerable biomedical research has been devoted to the development of pharmacological agents capable of alleviating the distressing symptoms of cardiac disorders. In particular, three general classes of drugs have found useful application in the prevention of angina during exercise and hence have increased the general physical working capacity of cardiac patients; the general classes are the cardiac glycosides, the vasodilators, and the beta-blocking agents. As early as 1939 Boje (56) discussed the possible use of digitalis, a cardiac glycoside, and nitroglycerin, a vasodilator, as potential ergogenic aids in sports. Although not specifically advocating beta-blocking agents as ergogenic aids for normal subjects, numerous reports have indicated increased physical performance ability in cardiac patients, while several have indicated either physiological or psychological effects which might enhance physical performance in normal subjects.

Aside from several of the vasodilators, these agents have not been employed as ergogenic aids in athletics. Nevertheless, rather extensive research has been conducted regarding their effect upon physical working capacity and associated physiological parameters, not only in cardiac cases but also in normal individuals. Thus, in light of the comment by Boje, it was deemed important to briefly allude to these agents and their effects upon human performance.

Digitalis and Other Cardiac Glycosides

Digitalis is a cardiotonic glycoside which is extracted from dried leaves of digitalis purpurea. It is used primarily in cases of coronary insufficiency and congestive heart failure. The exact mechanism is not completely understood, but the main pharmacological action results in an increase in the force of myocardial contraction without an increase in oxygen consumption. Thus, the mechanical efficiency of the heart is increased. Opinions are divided as to whether cardiotonic glycosides have any significant action on the peripheral vascular system, but peripheral circulation is improved due to the increased cardiac output.

Thus, if digitalis can increase the efficiency of the heart, its use might hypothetically be effectively applied to increase work capacity, as deVries (134) has indicated that the intrinsic functioning of the heart may be one of the limiting factors in human performance. Indeed, with cardiac patients, digitalization did elicit increases in physical working capacity (3). However, discussing the doping problem in athletics in 1939, Boje (56) indicated digitalis has no applicability to sports since it has no stimulating influence upon a healthy circulation. The results of contemporary research corroborate this statement.

Reports concerning the effect of cardiac glycosides upon physiological changes during submaximal exercise are contradictory. Williams and others (541) reported a decreased cardiac output in normal subjects during submaximal work following digoxin, while Nordstrom-Ohrberg (380) reported a reduced heart rate during low intensity exercise after digitalization. On the other hand, Rodman (432) and Seltzer (458) found no effect of digitalis on cardiac output during mild exercise. Russell and Reeves (441) and Bruce (70) reported no changes in submaximal heart rate following digoxin. Yu and others (556) found that 0.15 mg digoxin/10 kg did not affect ventilation, oxygen transport or oxygen debt during submaximal treadmill exercise.

In maximal or near-maximal tests, Muller and others (362) reported that digitalization over a period of eight weeks did not influence the physical working capacity of fifteen healthy women. Schroeder and his associates (450) reported similar findings following a prolonged digitalization. Russell and Reeves (441) studied the effects of digitalis upon heart rate, ventilation and oxygen uptake during maximal work capacity in normal subjects. In a well-designed repeated-measures study, ten subjects undertook a maximal treadmill test under three conditions: control, placebo, and following a digitalizing dose of digoxin of approximately 4.5 mg given over a three day period. The results indicated no significant changes in the physiological parameters or time to exhaustion. Thus, the authors concluded that the maximal capacity for aerobic work was not influenced by therapeutic doses of digoxin. In tests involving near-maximal work, Nordstrom-Ohrberg (380) indicated that digitalis did not affect heart rate, ventilation, oxygen uptake, stroke volume, cardiac output, lactate production, mechanical efficiency or calculated physical working capacity. Bruce and his colleagues (70) studied the effects of digoxin upon both static muscular endurance and dynamic exercise on a treadmill. Using a double-blind placebo design, they tested the effect of 3.5 to 5.0 mg digoxin upon four healthy men. Studying each subject several times on each test, they concluded that digoxin had no significant influence on either the sustained static endurance test or the bouts of fatiguing dynamic endurance on the treadmill. Cardiovascular responses during the treadmill exercise were not affected by digoxin.

Since digitalis increased the contractile force of the heart muscle, Hollmann and his associates (256) hypothesized it might exert an effect on skeletal muscles. Using ten sport students as subjects, they reported that digitalization over a ten day period, in contrast to a placebo, elicited no significant differences in the strength levels of major muscle groups.

Using rats as subjects, Aldinger (13) reported that digoxin, administered during a chronic training period involving swimming, had no significant augmenting effect on hypertrophy of the heart muscle.

In summary, unless the athlete is a cardiac patient involved in Masters competition, cardiac glycosides are not effective ergogenic aids for normal athletes.

Nitroglycerin and Other Vasodilators

Vasodilators can increase either coronary or peripheral blood flow in several ways. Some vasodilators may exert direct action on vascular smooth muscle, while others may serve as either alpha-adrenergic blocking agents or beta-adrenergic enhancing agents. Alpha-adrenergic blockade causes a marked vasodilation in the cutaneous vessels of the limbs, while beta-adrenergic stimulation increases blood supply primarily to the muscles.

The administration of nitroglycerin (glyceryl trinitrate) reduces the appearance of angina in cardiac patients undergoing exercise stress tests, and thus increases their physical working capacity. Parker and his colleagues (393) indicated the mechanism of its action may be twofold; nitroglycerin may decrease coronary vascular resistance and may also reduce the oxygen requirement of the left ventricle by reduced systemic vascular resistance through peripheral vasodilation. The other nitrites such as amyl and octyl nitrite have similar effects. Isosorbide nitrite is milder than nitroglycerin, but has a more prolonged action. There are other vasodilating drugs available such as nicotinic acid, nicotinyl tartrate (ronical), buphenine, and some tranquilizing agents, particularly rauwolfia alkaloids.

Nitroglycerin has been shown to increase coronary blood flow in normal men (334, 393) and may possibly facilitate peripheral blood flow due to its action on systemic blood vessels. Consequently, it has been used as an ergogenic aid in athletics. In 1939 Boje (56) stated that nitroglycerin may have been used in sport in an attempt to produce increased circulation capacity through vascular dilation, and in 1948 Asmussen and Boje (26) noted it had been used by professional marathon bicyclists because of its effect on the coronary vessels. More recently, Ulmark (512) indicated that international athletes, particularly those who need enormous amounts of blood to the leg muscles, take vasodilators in order to enhance performance capacity.

Experimentation regarding the effects of nitroglycerin and other vasodilators on maximal exercise performance is limited, and the following review includes all the studies uncovered.

The effect of various vasodilators upon selected cardiovascular changes during submaximal exercise has been investigated. Naughton and his colleagues (374) studied the effect of iso-sorbide dinitrate upon the heart rate response to a graded exercise test on the treadmill. Normal subjects chewed a 5.0 mg tablet twenty minutes prior to the test. In general, the heart rate was significantly lower under the drug condition, even at peak testing conditions. This finding would be indicative of a more efficient heart; however, the workload was probably submaximal as the mean peak heart rate was only 165. Testing ten healthy males at a workload of 600 kpm, Christensson and others (97) studied the effect of 0.5 mg nitroglycerin upon exercise cardiac output while in the supine and sitting position. There was no significant change in cardiac output while in the supine position, but a significant decrease occurred while sitting. On the contrary, Bousvaros and his colleagues (59) found that 10 mg dipyridamole, a potent vasodilator, increased cardiac output and stroke volume in nine healthy men during submaximal exercise. The exercise workload was only 300 kpm. Hoeschen and his colleagues (249) also noted an increased cardiac output during submaximal exercise following intake of nitroglycerin; both normal subjects and cardiac patients were tested. DeCrinis and others (129) indicated that the use of a vasodilator such as nylidrine hydrochloride could augment the blood flow to a muscle during exercise. Using a well-controlled design with three healthy subjects and seven patients with occlusive arterial disease, they noted that the intravenous administration of 7 mg nylidrine hydrochloride increased blood flow to the muscle during exercise above that which occurred during exercise alone. They concluded that the vasodilator apparently enhanced capacity of muscle vessels to respond to exercise.

If the above findings relative to increased cardiac output and blood flow could be extrapolated to a maximal exercise situation, then the vasodilators possibly would be able to increase maximal work capacity. Only a few reports have been found which studied this possibility.

In 1948, Asmussen and Boje (26) tested the influence of 1.0 mg nitroglycerin upon the capacity of three healthy athletes on two different work tasks. The exercises were performed on a bicycle ergometer and were designed to approximate energy expenditure in the 100 meter dash and 1500 meter run. The nitroglycerin had no effect upon performance; however, no placebo condition was utilized with the nitroglycerin testing. Ganslen and others (197) noted that 200 mg Recordil, an Italian vasodilator, increased the physical working capacity of two subjects four hours after ingestion; the criterion test was an all-out treadmill run to exhaustion. The authors noted that the absence of localized fatigue and pain in the legs supports the thesis that peripheral vasodilation occurred. However, no definite conclusion may be reached due to the small number of subjects.

Detry and Bruce (133) evaluated the effect of 0.4 mg nitroglycerin upon the maximal VO_2 of twelve healthy middle-aged subjects, thirty-two patients with angina, and twenty-three survivors of myocardial infarction free of angina. The nitroglycerin increased the maximal VO_2 in both patient groups, but not in the normal subjects. In a subsequent study, Bruce and others (71) reported that nitroglycerin increased the mean treadmill running time over thirty seconds in fifty male black workers. The maximal VO_2 increased from 29.7 to 31.5 ml/kg/minute;

it is evident by the max VO_2 values that the subjects were untrained men.

Although the physiological effects of the vasodilators may supply rationale for their use as ergogenic aids in endurance activities, no objective evidence is available with highly trained athletes to substantiate this hypothesis. Even though more blood may be delivered to a body part, this does not necessarily mean that the active muscles will be able to utilize the additional oxygen and nutrients.

Propranolol and Other Beta-Blocking Agents

In order to explain the differential effects of epinephrine and norepinephrine upon the various sympathetic effector organs in the body, two different receptor endings have been postulated; theoretically, the alpha-adrenergic endings are stimulated only by norepinephrine, whereas epinephrine can stimulate both alpha and beta-adrenergic endings. Beta-receptor stimulation induces increased force of myocardial contraction, cardio-acceleration, and vasodilation in the skeletal vasculature. As is obvious, these changes are beneficial during exercise and are normally elicited at the onset and duration of physical activity. Beta-blocking agents would negate these effects. Thus, it would appear that beta-blocking agents would not increase performance capacity, but would decrease it, especially endurance type events.

However, since propranolol and the other beta-blocking agents reduce the response of the heart to stress or exercise, it may be theorized that the cardiovascular system may be more efficient during physical activity. Barnard and Foss (35) reported that propranolol reduced the oxygen consumption and oxygen debts of dogs trained to run a given workload on a treadmill. They raised the interesting point that the dogs had greater mechanical efficiency under the propranolol condition. Thoren (504) studied the effects of 10 mg propranolol on exercise hemodynamics in eleven healthy boys, ages 9 to 11. He concluded that children can perform submaximal and maximal exercise after beta-adrenergic blockade with a significantly lower heart rate and blood lactate, indicating a better oxygen utilization by the muscle and greater aerobic work. The children also indicated the work seemed subjectively easier under the blockade. Blatter and Imhof (51) noted that beta-blocking produced a 34 percent decrease in the emotional heart rate response just prior to ski jumping. These findings may have implications for the use of propranolol in athletics, primarily for endurance events.

In cardiac patients who experience angina during exercise, numerous reports have indicated a significant increase in physical working capacity following the administration of propranolol or other agents. The beneficial effect is due to the decreased incidence of angina, which enables the patient to exercise longer. Goldbarg and others (207) noted propranolol did decrease the number of angina pectoris attacks, but did not significantly improve the treadmill exercise capacity in a group of cardiac patients. On the other hand, Furberg (193, 194), Sowton (489), Epstein (154), Hamer and Sowton (227), Dagenais (126), Coltart (106), Sealey (453), Astrom (28), Barbi (33), and Prichard and Gillam (410) all reported significant increases in efficiency or physical work capacity in cardiac patients following beta-blockade.

The important question for athletics, however, is concerned with the effects of beta-blockade on the normal subject, particularly one who is highly trained. Before considering the effects upon actual endurance capacity, the influence of beta-blocking agents upon adjustments to exercise will be reviewed.

The effect of beta-blocking agents upon exercise heart rate is consistent. Numerous reports (57, 66, 119, 123, 148, 168, 196, 329, 339, 340, 418, 455, 504) have indicated that both the submaximal and maximal heart rates are significantly reduced following beta-blockade. This effect would tend to produce a higher score on physical working capacity tests that predict PWC from the heart rate response to a standardized workload; examples are the PWC_{170} test of Sjostrand and Wahlund, and the Astrand-Rhyming nomogram. Furberg and Schmalensee (196) have substantiated this point; they reported a 15 percent increase in PWC_{170} in healthy subjects following the administration of 0.22 mg/kg propranolol. Results from submaximal tests such as these have many reservations in regards to predicting maximal performance capacity since the heart rate is only one component of the cardiac reserve.

Although several reports (123, 455) have noted a slight increase in exercise stroke volume, it must not be proportional to the decrease in heart rate as the submaximal and maximal cardiac output is reduced following beta-blockade (28, 119, 122, 123, 150, 152, 153, 194, 196, 418). Although the decrease in maximal cardiac output would appear to cause a concomitant decrease in max VO_2, the results of several reports are inconsistent. Epstein and his associates (153), using a tightly controlled experimental design, found that 0.15 mg/kg propranolol elicited a significant reduction in max VO_2 of seven normal subjects. On the other hand, with equally well-controlled experiments, Maksud and his associates (339, 340), Ekblom and Goldbarg (148), and Ekblom and others (150), reported no significant effect of propranolol upon max VO_2. The insignificant effect of propranolol on max VO_2 may be due to an increased a-v oxygen difference. Both Cronin (119) and Epstein (153) have reported increases in exercise a-v oxygen difference following propranolol, and Liesen (329) also noted a decrease in venous oxygen saturation. This result may follow from the finding of Knauf (302), who reported an increased, rather than a decreased, efficiency in muscular blood flow following propranolol. Thus, while the amount of blood leaving the heart during exercise may be decreased after propranolol administration, the tissues may extract more oxygen to meet their metabolic needs.

While the general results above indicate that max VO_2 is not affected by beta-blockade, the results appear otherwise for actual work output; although tentative, the findings suggest that propranolol may decrease physical work capacity.

In a summary primarily of his own research, Furberg (194) indicated that athletes experienced a slight decrease in endurance capacity at heavy work loads, probably because the reduced cardiac output during beta-blockade was not completely compensated for by other factors. This viewpoint would be supported by the findings of other reports. Epstein and others (153), using seven healthy males, reported that 0.15 mg/kg propranolol decreased maximal cardiac output and concomitantly produced a 40 percent decrease in time to exhaustion on an all-out tread-mill run. Ekblom and his associates (150) reported similar findings for fourteen healthy male nonathletes; maximal bicycle ergometer tests were used to evaluate the effect of 10 mg propranolol. Using dogs as subjects, Brzezinska and Nazar (72) reported that propranolol (0.25 mg/kg) and pronethalol (3 mg/kg) elicited a 42.8 percent decrease in endurance time in comparison to control conditions; the exercise was a test of prolonged endurance, as the time decreased from 203 to 120 minutes. They also found that the beta-blockade produced an earlier hypoglycemia, indicating that the adrenergic system is extremely important for the mobilization of energy-rich sub-strates during exercise. In a follow-up study, Nazar and his colleagues (375) studied the physiological mechanisms whereby beta-adrenergic blockade affected the capacity for prolonged muscular work. Propranolol (0.25 mg/kg) reduced the work capacity of dogs by 47.7 percent. Intravenous infusion of glucose restored the animals within 5 to 7 minutes and permitted an extension of the running time. Since the working capacity was restored when the glucose was infused into the systemic circulation, the authors concluded that the decisive factor con-trolling endurance in the dogs was the availability of energy substrate to the working muscles. They suggested that the im-pairment in physical performance was due to a more rapid depletion of muscle glycogen, since the beta-blocking agents inhibited the mobilization of lipids for energy use by the muscle.

On the other hand, several reports have noted no significant effect of beta-blocking agents upon maximal working capacity. Using a double-blind placebo design, Maksud and his colleagues (339) reported no detrimental effect of propranolol upon the endurance capacity of sixteen healthy young males subjected to a maximal bicycle ergometer test. They hypothesized that the cardiac depressant effects of propranolol are compensated for during exercise in normal subjects, and therefore PWC is not hampered. In a later study, Maksud and others (340) studied the effect of 0.44 mg/kg propranolol upon maximal endurance times on a multistage exercise task; eleven normal sedentary subjects were trained for twelve weeks and participated in both placebo and drug tests. Although the training program itself did elicit significant improvement in endurance times, the effect attributed to propranolol was insignificant when contrasted to the placebo, both before and after the conditioning period. However, it should be noted that the mean endurance time was 30 seconds less with propranolol than placebo, both before and after conditioning, although the difference was not statistically significant. Thoren (504) reported no significant effect of 10 mg propranolol upon the PWC to exhaustion of young boys, and Bollinger (57) noted no significant effects upon working capacity of healthy subjects.

Donald and his associates (142) studied the effect of beta-blockade on the racing performance of six normal greyhounds. Time to run five-sixteenths of a mile before and after blockade was the criterion test. The data revealed that 8 to 10 minutes after the administration of 1 to 2 mg/kg propranolol, the racing times were slightly slower with the drugs; but, the effect was of borderline significance. The authors suggested that blockade may be ineffective provided motivation is high and stimulation of the cardiac sympathetic nerves intense.

In one study (504), young male subjects indicated the exercise task seemed subjectively easier under beta-blockade, whereas Ekblom and Goldbarg (148) reported no significant subjective effects following propranolol in either submaximal or maximal exercise tests performed by nineteen healthy males.

In summary, whatever the mode of action of beta-blocking agents on maximal or prolonged work, it seems that these drugs are not useful as ergogenic aids in athletics. Although some studies have reported no significant decrease in performance capacity, others have noted deleterious effects and none have evinced beneficial effects.

CHAPTER 6

RESEARCH AND THE DOPING PROBLEM

Wհат is the solution to the drug problem in athletics—if any? The answer might be more readily attainable if we knew exactly how and what drugs consistently improve athletic performance. However, Csaky (120) indicated recently that the question as to whether the physical performance of well-trained healthy bodies can be increased by drugs cannot be answered with any degree of scientific assurance. Furthermore, one medical group indicated that the perfect legal definition of doping is impossible (354). Nevertheless, several authorities active in the field of sports medicine have widely divergent viewpoints concerning the doping problem. There are those who believe the use of drugs in athletics is scandalous and corrupts the basic purpose of sport, while others believe that if a drug is legal and possesses no serious health risk, then it should be made available to the athlete (204). These dichotomous viewpoints are probably due to individual interpretation of the available scientific data concerning doping. For example, dependent upon one's analysis and interpretation of the data from the extensive research project by Smith and Beecher (479, 480, 481), one could conclude either an enhancement effect or insignificant effect of amphetamines upon athletic performance.

Thus far the available research has not provided us with the facts in order to make sound decisions. If one considers the methodological differences in the studies reviewed in this book, some insight may be gained regarding the problem of making a valid interpretation and the futility of ascertaining whether or not a particular drug can enhance performance. Concerning drugs alone, there were differences in dosages, strength (e.g. Benzedrine vs Dexedrine®), absorption time or elapsed time prior to testing. Subjects included different species of animals, and humans of both sexes with divergent ages, health conditions, athletic backgrounds, and fitness levels. Double-blind placebo designs were not always utilized. Different types and sophistication of psychological and physiological tests were employed. In training studies with the anabolic steroids, exercise regimens varied considerably. Conditions in the studies ranged from controlled laboratory situations to diverse field studies; moreover, one is faced with the problem of extrapolating laboratory findings to field performance. Statistical techniques ranged from none to sophisticated covariance analyses. Other differences may be noted, and one should be cognizant of such factors when comparing the results of one study with another. Thus, to recapitulate, the current quilted approach to investigation of the doping problem precludes any valid statement relative to the effectiveness of doping.

If any sound decisions are to be made relative to drugs and sports, then a concerted research effort must be made in order to establish factual evidence. It would appear that if the public and the government wanted its sports programs to be based on the concept of equality and fair play, then the governments should undertake national, and probably international, research studies designed to evaluate the effectiveness of selected drugs. Factual data is needed on the effectiveness of various drugs, recommended dosages, adverse side effects, simple and effective detection methods to determine if a drug was used, costs, and other factors. The approach should probably be twofold, incorporating both laboratory and field experimentation. Laboratory experiments lend themselves to better experimental control, and the design and conduct of an experiment is only limited by the investigator's knowledge, imagination and available total environment for research. If an athletic conference, such as the Big Ten or Pacific Eight, would deem it important enough, possibly a controlled field research project could be conducted within the confines of the conference. The NCAA apparently considers the doping problem important, as they have recently conducted a survey of most college institutions relative to drug use among athletes. One step further might involve them in actual scientific investigations to ascertain, possibly once and for all, the effectiveness of doping.

It is to be hoped that some type of coordinated effort would be developed to research the doping problem; if not, individual research is still valuable, for all information, if appropriately collected, may be useful in answering the doping question Therefore, individual research projects are still encouraged.

RESEARCH CONSIDERATIONS

For the interested investigator, there are several points of experimental protocol and methodology which should be considered when studying the effects of drugs on human performance.

Since pharmacological agents are being introduced into humans, it is imperative that the experimentation be approved and supervised by medical personnel who are aware of the actions of the specific drugs during physical activity. Subjects should undergo medical examinations prior to experimentation with particular attention directed towards the detection of conditions which could be aggravated by the administration of the drug under consideration. In this light, informed consent forms should be developed specifying the purpose and nature of the experiment, drugs consumed, and possible adverse effects. Every attempt should be made to inform the subjects of their role in the experiment and to answer any questions they may have relative to their participation. Although this may complicate the application of a truly double-blind investigation, ethical considerations supercede methodological precepts.

The administration of the drug relative to dosage, pharmacological effect, and subsequent testing of physical performance should be well planned. In most cases, dosages should be based on body weight and, if possible, variant dosages should be assigned in order to evaluate a trend effect and dose response relationships. For example, alcohol could be administered as a placebo, small, moderate, or large dose. The alcohol may be beneficial at a small dose and detrimental at larger levels; thus, the pharmacological action relative to physical activity may be dose dependent. Time dependent factors may also be important considerations. Certain drugs may elicit maximal benefit immediately after ingestion, while others might exert their desired, or possibly detrimental, effects some time afterwards. Thus, the time for testing of physical performance should be based on the interaction of the dose response and time dependent factors of the drug in question.

Certain experimental designs are more appropriate than others. Whenever feasible, repeated measures designs should be used, for they allow for control of intersubject differences. In effect, each subject serves as his own control, and variability due to differences in the average responsiveness of subjects is eliminated from experimental error. Placebo doses can easily be incorporated into this design. However, if a practice or training effect may occur related to the performance of the criterion test, then the order of the administration of drugs should be counterbalanced either randomly or by Latin square techniques. Although a strict double-blind procedure is impossible under the conditions of informed consent, the use of several different dosages and a placebo, and the administration of the dosages by someone other than the principal investigator, may satisfy the principles underlying the concept of double-blind experimentation. The subject may know he is receiving a drug, but he will not be aware of when he is receiving the variant dosages or the placebo, and the principal investigator will not know what dosage has been given. If these conditions prevail, they will help to eliminate such experimental artifact as the halo effect, Rosenthal effect, Hawthorne effect, and demand characteristics, which ofttimes confound doping research.

Generalizations are limited by the nature of the sampling criteria and criterion measure used. Results obtained from a sample of students obtained from a required college physical education class may not necessarily apply to conditioned athletes. Consequently, whenever possible, athletes who would supposedly benefit from the use of a particular drug should be incorporated in the investigation. For example, blood doping (blood reinjection) has been hypothesized to benefit long distance runners; hence, this class of athletes should be utilized in experimentation with blood doping. One should also be concerned with the validity of the criterion test, especially if it is a laboratory test. If a subject is administered a drug and is able to run for a longer period of time on a treadmill, this does not necessarily mean that he will run faster on a track. Thus, specificity of performance should be attained whenever possible.

In all out performance, both psychological and physiological variables determine the limits of man's capacity. Yet, in most studies involving the effect of drugs on athletic performance only physiological variables are tested and little attention is devoted to the psychological domain. A noted exception is the three part report on amphetamines by Smith and Beecher (479, 480, 481). Morgan (360) suggested that in future research a multivariate psychobiological approach would be useful, as it would reveal interaction of drug effects on both physiological and psychological factors in human performance.

Thus, it goes unsaid that careful preplanning is especially necessary in doping experimentation with human subjects. Animal studies are useful, but it is difficult many times to extrapolate the findings to humans.

EDUCATION AGAINST DOPING

The solution to the doping problem is education, but it is not a simple one. At the present time, on the basis of this literature review, there appears to be no sound experimental evidence to substantiate a consistent effect of any drug as an ergogenic aid for athletic performance. Even though this concept of the ineffectiveness of doping could be communicated to athletes, they would probably maintain the belief that a magic potion exists which will enable them to perform more effectively. One need only observe American television for one Saturday morning in order to comprehend part of the foundation for this belief. Within a four hour time span the child is bombarded with information, artistically and educationally well designed, that Popeye's spinach, supervitamins, energy loaded cereal, power candy bars, or superman sneakers will instantly produce a super-boy or supergirl. Along with these commercials aimed specifically at the preadolescent population, the child is also exposed to numerous advertisements extolling the virtues of various drug preparations for instant relief from pain, neuritis, neuralgia, and even tired blood. Underlying most of these commercials is the fact that if the product is consumed, the individual will be more energetic and capable of being more active, usually within a very short period of time. It is highly conceivable that during the 15,000 hours of television the average child watches through late adolescence, information such as this may have a bearing on the athlete's attitudes towards drug use in sports. In addition, once the child enters the world of athletics, he is usually exposed to cherished beliefs that have survived the years and still permeate junior and senior high school locker rooms; meat is energy food, use wheat germ oil, honey gives you quick energy—are only a few examples of comments the young athlete hears which may generate, or reinforce, the concept that some substances enhance performance. The athletic training room may be stocked with dextrose tablets, vitamin C tablets, butterfly tablets, as well as other supplements with the dubious, although explicitly adver-tised, purpose to energize or powerize the athlete. Although there may be some sound medical reasons for the use of these substances, the coach or trainer who indicates to his athletes that these compounds will facilitate performance may perpetuate belief in the magic potion. As a side point, but one which reflects back on the problems associated with the definition of doping, several sports medicine authorities (120, 309) have indicated the use of placebos constitutes doping, if the athlete is made to believe it is an active substance. Thus, the coach who admin-isters harmless dextrose tablets to his athletes, with the sugges-tion that they will charge him wih energy, may elicit the well known placebo effect; although this may or may not be doping, it may affect the athlete's attitudes and behavior towards doping.

In addition to coaches and trainers, Francesconi (181) also indicated that the behavior of the team physician may have a tremendous impact on the athlete's attitude towards doping, and cautioned him to be careful in the use of drugs with athletes.

Prokop (413) indicated that some physicians administer drugs to athletes with astonishing liberality, hoping to provide him with that winning edge.

The educational process against doping is not only the domain of those involved in sports. Education about drugs in general should begin at home and continue through the school years. If the child can obtain sound knowledge and develop healthy attitudes about the values and dangers of drugs, then chances are his behavior will follow accordingly. If doping is to be eliminated, this behavior needs to be reinforced by those involved in the educational and administrative aspects of athletics. Of prime importance is knowledge concerning health hazards of drug use in athletics, and communication of this to the athlete.

Consequently, if the use of drugs in sports is to be eradicated, it will take the cooperation of parents, teachers, coaches, athletes, trainers, physicians, athletic governing bodies, and the sports press. In addition, the scientific data need to be provided by competent investigators. The goal is a distant one, but worthy of pursuing.

BIBLIOGRAPHY

1. AAHPER: Report of a national conference: Value in sports. Washington, American Association for Health, Physical Education and Recreation, 1963.
2. AAHPER: Clarke, K. (Ed.): *Drugs and the Coach*. Washington, American Association for Health, Physical Education and Recreation, 1972.
3. Aberg, H., and others: The effect of digitalis on the heart rate during exercise in patients with atrial fibrillation. *Acta Med Scand, 191*:441-45, 1972.
4. Adamson, G., and Finley, S.: The effects of two psycho-stimulant drugs on muscular performance in male athletes. *Ergonomics, 8*:237-41, 1965.
5. Adamson, G., and Finley, S.: A comparison of the effects of varying dose levels of oxypertine on mood and physical performance of trained athletes.*Br J Psychiatry, 112*:1177-80, 1966.
6. Adolph, J.: *The effects of ethyl alcohol on physical performance.* Unpublished doctoral dissertation, The Ohio State University, 1969.
7. Ahlborg, B., and others: Muscle glycogen and muscle electrolytes during prolonged physical exercise. *Acta Physiol Scand, 70*:129-42, 1967.
8. Ahlborg, B., and others: Effect of potassium-magnesium-aspartate on the capacity for prolonged exercise in man. *Acta Physiol Scand, 74*:238-45, 1968.
9. Aksnes, E.: Effect of small dosages of alcohol upon performance in a link trainer. *J Aviat Med, 25*:680, 1954.
10. Albrecht, H., and Albrecht, E.: Ergometric, rheographic, reflexographic and electrocardiographic tests at altitude and effect of drugs on human physical performance. *Fed Proc, 28*:1262-67, 1969.
11. Alcohol metabolism during rest and exercise. *Nutr Rev, 24*:239-40, 1966.
12. Alcohol—The latest teen drug. *Newsweek*, March 5, 1973.
13. Aldinger, E.: Effects of digitoxin on the development of cardiac hypertrophy in the rat subjected to chronic exercise. *Am J Cardiol, 25*:339-43, 1970.
14. Alles, G., and Feigen, G.: The influence of benzedrine on work-decrement and patellar reflex. *Am J Physiol, 136*:392-400, 1942.

15. Altland, P., and Highman, B.: Effects of polycythemia and altitude hypoxia on rat heart and exercise tolerance. *Am J Physiol, 221*: 388-93, 1971.

16. Amphetamine and athletic performance. *Med J Aust, 46*:728-29, 1959.

17. Anabolic steroids and athletics. *Br Med J, 1*:104, 1971.

18. Anderson, J., and Brown, C.: A study of the effects of smoking upon grip strength and recuperation from local muscular fatigue. *Res Quart, 22*:102-8, 1951.

19. Androgenic and anabolic hormones. *Med Lett Drugs Ther, 8*:35-36, 1966.

20. Ariel, G.: *The effect of anabolic steroids on reflex components and skeletal muscle contractile force.* Paper presented at the 19th Annual Meeting, American College of Sports Medicine, Philadelphia, May 1, 1972.

21. Ariel, G.: Residual effect of anabolic steroid upon muscular force. *Med Sci Sports, 5*:59, 1973.

22. Ariel, G., and Saville, W.: The effect of anabolic steroids on reflex components. *Med Sci Sports, 4*:120-23, 1972.

23. Ariel, G., and Saville, W.: Anabolic steroids: the physiological effects of placebos. *Med Sci Sports, 4*:124-26, 1972.

24. Ariens, E.: Centrally-active drugs and performance in sports. *Schweiz Z Sportmed, 13*:77-98, 1965.

25. Asdell, S.: Sex steroid hormones and voluntary exercise in rats. *J Reprod Fertil, 3*:26-32, 1962.

26. Asmussen, E., and Boje, O.: The effects of alcohol and some drugs on the capacity for work. *Acta Physiol Scand, 15*:109-18, 1948.

27. Astrand, P., and Rodahl, K.: *Textbook of Work Physiology.* New York, McGraw-Hill, 1970.

28. Astrom, H.: Haemodynamic effects of beta-adrenergic blockade. *Br Heart J, 30*:44-49, 1968.

29. Balke, B., and others: Work capacity after blood donation. *J Appl Physiol, 7*:231-38, 1954.

30. Balke, B., and others: Altitude and maximum performance in work and sports activity. *JAMA, 194*:646-49, 1965.

31. Balke, B., and others: Maximum performance capacity at sea-level and at moderate altitude before and after training at altitude. *Schweiz Z Sportmed, 14*:106-16, 1966.

32. Banister, E.: Blood levels of adrenergic amines during exercise. *J Appl Physiol, 33*:674-6, 1972.

33. Barbi, G., and others: The effect of a new beta-blocking drug (Butidrine) on some biohumoral indices, liver and kidney function and exercise tolerance. *Panminerva Med, 11*:372-7, 1969.

34. Bard, P.: *Medical Physiology,* St. Louis, Mosby, 1960.

35. Barnard, R., and Foss, M.: Oxygen debt: effect of beta-adrenergic blockade on the lactacid and alactacid components. *J Appl Physiol, 27*:813-16, 1969.

36. Barnes, R., and others: Effects of exercise and administration of aspartic acid on blood ammonia in the rat. *Am J Physiol, 207*: 1242-46, 1964.

37. Bartak, K., and Skranc, O.: Effect of psychoton and dexfenmetrazin on maximal physical performance. *Physiol Bohemoslov, 19*:117-21, 1970.

38. Bartak, K., and Skranc, O.: The influence of psychoton and dexfenmetrazin on the duration of heavy work. *Int Z Angew Physiol, 30*:95-104, 1972.

39. Bass, D., and Jacobson, E.: Effects of salicylate on acclimitization to work in the heat. *J Appl Physiol, 20*:70-2, 1965.

40. Bastide, R.: *Doping.* Paris, Raoul Solar, 1970.

41. Battig, K.: Das Schwimmen von Ratten durch einen Wasserkanal methodische und pharmakilogische Einflusse auf Leistung und Ermudung. *Helv Physiol Acta, 19*:384-98, 1961.

42. Battig, K.: The effect of training and amphetamine on the endurance and velocity of swimming performance of rats. *Psychopharmacologia, 4*:15-27, 1963.

43. Battig, K.: Modellversuche an der Ratte uber die Art der Amphetaminwirkung bei verschieden Strukturierten Leistungen. *Schweiz Z Sportmed, 3*:99-116, 1965.

44. Battig, K.: Die Wirkung von Nikotin auf die Schwimmausdauer Testgewohnter Ratten. *Z Praventivmed, 13*:111-21, 1968.

45. Battig, K.: The effect of nicotine on the swimming speed of pretrained rats through a water alley. *Psychopharmacologia, 15*:19-27, 1969.

46. Baugh, R.: *The use and misuse of drugs among high school athletes.* American School Health Convention, Chicago, October 8, 1971.

47. Becker, W.: Doping—an Olympic problem. *Ther Ggw, 111*:1184-93, 1972.

48. Beckett, A., and others: Routine detection and identification in urine of stimulants and other drugs, some of which may be used to modify performance in sport. *J Pharm Pharmacol, 19*:273-94, 1967.

49. Begbie, G.: The effects of alcohol and of varying amounts of visual information on a balancing test. *Ergonomics, 9*:325-33, 1966.

50. Berne, R., and Levy, M.: *Cardiovascular Physiology.* St. Louis, Mosby, 1967.

51. Blatter, K., and Imhof, P.: The role of the adrenergic beta-receptors in emotional tachycardia; radiotelemetric studies on ski jumpers. *Schweiz Z Sportmed, 17*:131-49, 1969.

52. Blomqvist, G., and others: Acute effects of ethanol ingestion on the response to submaximal and maximal exercise in man. *Circulation,* 42:463-70, 1970.

53. Blood doping. *Track and Field News.* Los Altos, November, 1971.

54. Bobo, W.: Effects of alcohol upon maximum oxygen uptake, lung ventilation, and heart rate. *Res Quart,* 43:1-6, 1972.

55. Body building by drugs. *Br Med J,* 4:310-11, 1967.

56. Boje, O.: Doping. *Bull Health Org League of Nations,* 8:439-69, 1939.

57. Bollinger, A., and others: Pulsfrequenz und Leistungsfahigkeit vor und nach Beta-Rezeptoren-Blockade durch Propranolol. *Schweiz Med Wochenschr,* 95:1075-79, 1965.

58. Borg, G., and others: Changes in physical performance induced by amphetamines and amobarbital. *Psychopharmacologia,* 26:10-18, 1972.

59. Bousvaros, G., and others: Haemodynamic effects of dipyridamole at rest and during exercise in healthy subjects. *Br Heart J,* 28:331-34, 1966.

60. Bouton, J.: *Ball Four.* New York, World Pub, 1970.

61. Bouvet, A.: Clinical trial of pyridoscorbine in sport medicine: investigation of its refreshing and detoxication action (ski contest). *Gaz Med France,* 72:2571-3, 1965.

62. Bovet, D., and Amorico, L.: Effect of amphetamine on a conditioned avoidance reaction during prolonged exercise. *C R Acad Sci,* 256:3901-4, 1963.

63. Bowers, R., and Reardon, J.: Effects of methadrostenolone (Dianabol) on strength development and aerobic capacity. *Med Sci Sports,* 4:54, 1972.

64. Brashear, R., and Ross, J.: Effect of dipyridamole and propranolol on pulmonary diffusing capacity during rest and exercise. *Amer Rev Respir Dis,* 98:1048-51, 1968.

65. Brick, I., and others: Effects of propranolol on peripheral vessels in man. *Amer J Cardiol,* 18:329-32, 1966.

66. Brick, I., and others: Comparison of the effects of I. C. I. 50172 and propranolol on the cardiovascular responses to adrenaline, isoprenaline and exercise. *Br J Pharmacol,* 34:127-40, 1968.

67. Broun, H.: The 1984 Olympics. *Newsweek,* March 5, 1973.

68. Brown, B., and Pilch, A.: The effects of exercise and Dianabol upon selected performances and physiological parameters in the male rat. *Med Sci Sports,* 4:159-65, 1972.

69. Brown, C., and Searle, L.: The effect of variation in the dose of benzedrine sulfate on the activity of white rats. *J Exp Psychol,* 22:555-64, 1938.

70. Bruce, R., and others: The effects of digoxin on fatiguing static and dynamic exercise in man. *Clin Sci,* 34:29-42, 1968.

71. Bruce, R., and others: Divergent effects of antihypertensive therapy on cardiovascular responses and left ventricular function during upright exercise. *Am J Cardiol, 30*:768-74, 1972.

72. Brzezinska, A., and Nazar, K.: Effect of beta-adrenergic blockade on exercise metabolism in the dog. *Arch Int Physiol Biochem, 78*: 883-93, 1970.

73. Bugyi, G.: *The effects of moderate doses of caffeine on fatigue parameters of the forearm flexor muscles.* Unpublished master's thesis, University of Maryland, College Park, 1969.

74. Bujas, Z., and Petz, B.: Utjecaj fenamina na ekonomicnost staticnog rada. *Archiv za Higijenv Rada, 6*:205-8, 1955.

75. Bujas, Z., and others: Effect of some pharmacological agents on the efficiency of repeated physical performances. *Archiv za Higijenv Rada, 11*:261-87, 1960.

76. Burch, G.: The effect of ingestion of ethyl alcohol, wine and beer on the myocardium of mice. *Am J Cardiol, 27*:522-28, 1971.

77. Burger, A.: *Drugs Affecting the Nervous System.* New York, Dekker, 1968.

78. Burn, J.: Action of nicotine on the heart. *Ann NY Acad Sci, 90*:70-73, 1960.

79. Burt, J.: *The significance of athletic competition in the life of the mind.* Paper presented at the National AAHPER Convention, Minneapolis, April 13, 1973.

80. Buskirk, E., and others: Maximal performance at altitude and on return from altitude in conditioned runners. *J Appl Physiol, 23*:259, 1967.

81. Buterbaugh, G.: The use of drugs in athletics. *Md State Med J, 19*:69-70, 1970.

82. Cameron, J., and others: Effects of amphetamines on moods, emotions and motivation. *J Psychol, 61*:93-121, 1965.

83. Campos, F., and others: Some conditions affecting the capacity for prolonged muscular work. *Am J Physiol, 87*:680-701, 1928.

84. Carlsson, C., and others: Noradrenaline in human blood plasma and urine during exercise in patients receiving large doses of chlorpromazine. *Acta Pharmacol, 25*:97-106, 1967.

85. Carpenter, J.: The effects of caffeine and alcohol on simple visual reaction time. *J Comp Physiol Psychol, 52*:491-96, 1959.

86. Carpenter, J.: Effects of alcohol on some psychological processes. *Q J Stud Alcohol, 23*:274-314, 1962.

87. Cartoni, G., and Cavalli, A.: Detection of doping by thin layer and gas chromatography. *J Chromatogr, 37*:158-61, 1968.

88. Casner, S., and others: Anabolic steroid effects on body composition in normal young men. *J Sports Med Phys Fitness, 11*:98-103, 1971.

89. Catton, B.: *The Army of the Potomac: Mr. Lincoln's Army.* Garden City, Doubleday, 1951.

90. Centonza, D., and others: Coffee in the diet of the sportsman. *Minerva Med, 63*:3351-5, 1972.

91. Chaterjee, A., and others: Influence of methylamphetamine on blood lactic acid following exercise. *Jap J Pharmacol, 20*:170-2, 1970.

92. Cheney, R.: Comparative effect of caffeine per se and a caffeine beverage (coffee) upon the reaction time in normal young adults. *J Pharmacol, 53*:304-13, 1935.

93. Cheney, R.: Reaction time behavior after caffeine and coffee consumption. *J Exp Psychol, 19*:357-69, 1936.

94. Chenowith, L., and Selkirk, T.: *School Health Problems.* Des Moines, Appleton, 1953.

95. Chevalier, R., and others: Circulatory and ventilatory effects of exercise in smokers and non-smokers. *J Appl Physiol, 18*:357-60, 1963.

96. Chidsey, C., and others: Influence of syrosingopine on the cardiovascular response to acute hypoxemia and exercise. *Circ Res, 9*:989-95, 1961.

97. Christensson, B., and others: Haemodynamic effects of nitroglycerin in normal subjects during supine and sitting exercise. *Br Heart J, 31*:80-2, 1969.

98. Chroscielewski, E.: Pharmacological doping in sports. *Pol Tyg Lek, 24*:188-91, 1969.

99. Clarke, E.: Dope and doping. *Med Sci Law, 9*:218-23, 1969.

100. Clarke, K.: Quackery and sports. *Ohio Med J, 64*:913-20, 1968.

101. Clarke, K.: Drugs, sports and doping. *J Maine Med Assoc, 61*:55-8, 1970.

102. Cobley, J.: *Track and Field News,* May 16, 1971.

103. Cochran, W., and others: A reply. *JAMA, 177*:348, 1959.

104. Cohen, S.: *The Drug Dilemma.* New York, McGraw-Hill, 1969.

105. Collier, H.: Aspirin. *Sci Am, 209*:96-108, 1963.

106. Coltart, D.: Comparison of effects of propranolol and practolol on exercise tolerance in angina pectoris. *Br Heart J, 33*:62-4, 1971.

107. Consolazio, C., and others: Effects of aspartic acid salts (Mg+K) on physical performance of men. *J Appl Physiol, 19*:257-61, 1964.

108. Cooper, D.: Drugs and the athlete. *JAMA, 221*:1007-11, 1972.

109. Cooper, K.: Effects of cigarette smoking on endurance performance. *JAMA, 203*:189-92, 1968.

110. Coopersmith, S.: The effects of alcohol on reaction to affective stimuli. *Q J Stud Alcohol, 25*:459-75, 1964.

111. Cooter, G.: *The effect of amphetamine on maximal endurance.* Paper presented at the National AAHPER Convention, Houston, Texas, 1972.

112. Cornacchia, H., and others: *Drugs in the Classroom.* St. Louis, Mosby, 1973.

113. Costello, C.: The effect of stimulant and depressant drugs on physical persistence. *Am J Psychol, 76*:698-700, 1963.

114. Council on Drugs, AMA: New drugs and developments in therapeutics: potassium and magnesium aspartates (Spartase). *JAMA, 183*:362, 1963.

115. Coutts, C.: Freedom in sport. *Quest, 10*:70, 1968.

116. Cox, B., and Toohey, J.: Anabolic steroids and athletes. *Scholastic Coach, 40*:50, January, 1971.

117. Craig, A.: Limitations of the human organism. Analysis of world records and Olympic performance. *JAMA, 205*:734-40, 1968.

118. Crancer, A., and others: Comparison of the effects of marijuana on simulated driving performance. *Science, 164*:851-54, 1969.

119. Cronin, R.: Hemodynamic and metabolic effects of beta-adrenergic blockade in exercising dogs. *J Appl Physiol, 22*:211-16, 1967.

120. Csaky, T.: Doping. *J Sports Med Phys Fitness, 12*:117-23, 1972.

121. Cuiffardi, T.: Dosis de alcaloides que ingieren los habituados a la coca; nuevas observaciones. *Rev Farmacol y Med Exptl, 2*:216-31, 1949.

122. Cumming, G., and Carr, W.: Hemodynamic response to exercise after propranolol in normal subjects. *Can J Physiol Pharmacol, 44*:465-74, 1966.

123. Cumming, G., and Carr, W.: Hemodynamic response to exercise after beta-adrenergic and parasympathetic blockade. *Can J Physiol Pharmacol, 45*:813-19, 1967.

124. Cuthbertson, D., and Knox, J.: The effects of amphetamine on the fatigued subject. *J Physiol, 106*:43-58, 1947.

125. Cutinelli, L., and others: Protection by ornithine-aspartate of the effects of physical exercise. *Arzneim Forsch, 20*:1064-7, 1970.

126. Dagenais, G., and others: Exercise tolerance in patients with angina pectoris. Daily variation and effects of erythrityl tetranitrate, propranolol and alprenolol. *Am J Cardiol, 28*:10-16, 1971.

127. Danysz, A., and others: The influence of 2-dimethylaminethanol (DMAE) on the mental and physical efficiency in man. *Activ Nerv Sup, 9*:417, 1967.

128. Danzinger, R., and Cumming, G.: Effects of chlorthiazide on working capacity of normal subjects. *J Appl Physiol, 19*:636-8, 1964.

129. DeCrinis, K., and others: Vascular effects of nylidrine hydrochloride during exercise. *Proc Soc Exp Biol Med, 102*:29-31, 1959.

130. DeCristofaro, D., and Liu, C.: The haemodynamics of cardiac tamponade and blood volume overload in dogs. *Cardiovas Res, 3*:292-98, 1969.

131. Dennig, H.: Uber Steigerung der korperlichen Leistungsfahigkeit durch Eingriffe in den Sauerbasenhaushalt. *Deutsch Med Wochenschr, 63*:733-36, 1937.

132. Dennig, H., and others: Effect of acidosis and alkalosis upon capacity for work. *J Clin Invest, 9*:601-13, 1931.

133. Detry, J., and Bruce, R.: Effects of nitroglycerin on maximal oxygen uptake and exercise electrocardiogram in coronary disease. *Circulation, 43*:155-63, 1971.

134. deVries, H.: *Physiology of Exercise for Physical Education and Athletics.* Dubuque, Brown, 1966.

135. deVries, H., and Adams, G.: Electromyographic comparison of single doses of exercise and meprobamate as to effects on muscular relaxation. *Am J Phys Med, 51*:130-41, 1972.

136. deWijn, J., and others: Haemoglobin, packed cell volume, serum iron and iron binding capacity of selected athletes during training. *J Sports Med Phys Fitness, 11*:42-51, 1971.

137. Dill, D., and others: Alkalosis and the capacity for work. *J Biol Chem, 97*:58-59, 1932.

138. Dill, D., and others: Studies in muscular activity. *J Physiol, 77*:49-62, 1932.

139. Dirix, A.: The doping problem at the Tokyo and Mexico City Olympic Games. *J Sport Med, 6*:183-6, 1966.

140. Doctor, R., and Perkins, R.: The effects of ethyl alcohol on autonomic and muscular responses in humans. *Q J Stud Alcohol, 22*:374-86, 1961.

141. Doll, P.: Medicine and doping. *Med Leg Domm Corpor, 2*:228-35, 1969.

142. Donald, D., and others: Effect of beta-adrenergic receptor blockade on racing performance of greyhounds with normal and with denervated hearts. *Circ Res, 22*:127-34, 1968.

143. Dope—the hidden hang up in sports. *This Week Magazine*, September 8, 1965.

144. Downey, J., and Darling, R.: Effect of salicylates on elevation of body temperature during exercise. *J Appl Physiol, 17*:323-5, 1962.

145. Downey, J., and Darling, R.: Effects of salicylates on exercise metabolism. *J Appl Physiol, 17*:665-8, 1962.

146. Eagle, E., and others: Influence of cortico-adrenal extracts on energy output. *Am J Physiol, 102*:707-13, 1932.

147. Eckstein, J., and Abboud, F.: Circulatory effects of sympathomimetic amines. *Am Heart J, 63*:119-35, 1962.

148. Ekblom, B., and Goldbarg, A.: The influence of physical training and other factors on the subjective rating of perceived exertion. *Acta Physiol Scand, 83*:399-406, 1971.

149. Ekblom, B., and others: Response to exercise after blood loss and reinfusion. *J Appl Physiol, 33*:175-80, 1972.

150. Ekblom, B., and others: Effects of atropine and propranolol on the oxygen transport system during exercise in man. *Scand J Clin Lab Invest, 30*:35-42, 1972.

151. Ekelund, L., and others: Central hemodynamic effects in man of intravenous d-alprenolol during rest and exercise. *Eur J Clin Pharmacol, 3*:198-203, 1971.

152. Ekstrom-Jodal, B., and others: The effect of adrenergic-receptor blockage on coronary circulation in man during work. *Acta Med Scand, 191*:245-8, 1972.

153. Epstein, S., and others: Effects of beta-adrenergic blockade on the cardiac response to maximal and submaximal exercise in man. *J Clin Invest, 44*:1745-53, 1965.

154. Epstein, S., and others: Angina pectoris: pathophysiology, evaluation, and treatment. *Ann Intern Med, 75*:263-96, 1971.

155. Evans, W., and Caldwell, L.: The effects of the potassium and magnesium salts of dl-aspartic acid on human fatigue and recovery. *U S Army Med Res Lab Rep, 550*:5p, 16 Aug, 1962.

156. Eysenck, H., and others: The effect of stimulant and depressant drugs on continuous work. *J Mental Sci, 103*:645-49, 1957.

157. Fahey, T., and Brown, H.: *Effects of anabolic steroids plus weight training on normal males—a double blind study.* Paper presented at 19th Annual Meeting, American College of Sports Medicine, Philadelphia, May 1, 1972.

158. Fallis, N., and others: Effect of potassium and magnesium aspartates on athletic performance. *JAMA, 185*:129, 1963.

159. Falls, H.: *Exercise Physiology,* New York, Acad Pr, 1968.

160. Feldscher, D.: *Effect of anabolic steroid (oxandrolone) on endurance, body weight, specific gravity, and percentage of body fat in male rats.* Unpublished master's thesis, University of Maryland, College Park, 1972.

161. Ferguson, T., and others: Effect of blood and saline infusion on ventricular end diastolic pressure, stroke work, stroke volume and cardiac output in the open and closed chest dog. *Circ Res, 1*:62-68, 1953.

162. Fewings, J., and others: The effects of ethyl alcohol on the blood vessels of the hand and forearm in man. *Br J Pharmacol Chemother, 27*:93-106, 1966.

163. Fischbach, E.: The doping problem from a new point of view. *Munchen Med Wochenschr, 107*:1783-6, 1965.

164. Fischbach, E.: Coffee and sports. *Minerva Med, 61*:4367-9, 1970.

165. Fischbach, E.: Problems of doping. *Med Monatsschr, 26*:377-81, 1972.

166. Fisher, A., and others: *The effect of acetylsalicylic acid ingestion upon maximal oxygen uptake, maximal running time, and oxygen debt of highly trained endurance athletes.* Paper presented at National AAHPER Convention, Houston, Texas, March 25, 1972.

167. Fleming, D.: On living in a biological revolution. *The Atlantic Monthly,* February, 1969.

168. Floor-Wieringa, A., and others: Effect of beta-adrenergic blocking drugs on the heart rate during submaximal exercise. *Eur J Pharmacol, 10*:303-10, 1970.
169. Flory, C., and Gilbert, J.: The effects of benzedrine sulfate and caffeine citrate on the efficiency of college students. *J Appl Physiol, 27*:121-34, 1943.
170. Foldes, F., and others: The influence of exercise on the neuromuscular activity of relaxant drugs. *Can Anaesth Soc J, 8*:118-27, 1961.
171. Foldi-Borcsok, E., and others: Improvement of physical capacity in the swimming test by an unspecified stimulant. *Arzneim Forsch, 21*:1735-7, 1971.
172. Folle, L., and others: Hemodynamic response to exercise after beta-adrenergic blockade in normal and labile hypertensive patients. *Cardiology, 55*:105-13, 1970.
173. Foltz, E., and others: The use of double work periods in the study of fatigue and the influence of caffeine on recovery. *Am J Physiol, 136*:79, 1942.
174. Foltz, E., and others: The influence of amphetamine (benzedrine) sulfate and caffeine on the performance of rapidly exhausting work by untrained subjects. *J Lab Clin Med, 28*:601-3, 1943.
175. Foltz, E., and others: The influence of amphetamine (benzedrine) sulfate, d-desoxyephedrine hydrochloride (pervitan), and caffeine upon work output and recovery when rapidly exhausting work is done by trained subjects. *J Lab Clin Med, 28*:603-6, 1943.
176. Forney, R., and others: Measurement of attentive motor performance after alcohol. *Percept Mot Skills, 19*:151-54, 1964.
177. Fowler, W.: The facts about ergogenic aids and sports performance. *J Amer Assn Health Phys Educ and Rec, 40*:37-42, 1969.
178. Fowler, W., and others: Effect of an anabolic steroid on physical performance of young men. *J Appl Physiol, 20*:1038-40, 1965.
179. Fowler, W., and others: Ineffective treatment of muscular dystrophy with an anabolic steroid and other measures. *New Engl J Med, 272*:875-82, 1965.
180. Fox, M., and others: Oxandrolone: a potent anabolic steroid of novel chemical configuration. *J Clin Endocrinol Metab, 22*:921-24, 1962.
181. Francesconi, A.: Medicine in sport: doping. *Ann Med Nav, 67*:772-81, 1962.
182. Frankenhaeuser, M., and Myrsten, A.: Performance decrement after intake of meprobamate as a function of task difficulty and learning level. *Percept Motor Skills, 27*:839-43, 1968.
183. Freed, D., and others: Anabolic steroids in athletics. *Br Med J, 3*:761, 1972.
184. Frenkl, R., and others: Effects and elimination of prednisolone in physically trained and untrained subjects. *Int Z Angew Physiol, 28*:131-4, 1970.

185. Frey, H.: Anabolic steroids for athletics. *Tidsskr Nor Laegeforen,* 91:289-90, 1971.

186. Frey, U.: Doping. *Med Welt, 31*:1590-2, 1960.

187. Frommel, E., and others: On the action of nikethamide (Coramine) on the centers of thermoregulation and on muscular efficiency. *Helv Physiol Pharmacol Acta, 21*:10-6, 1963.

188. Fruehan, A., and Frawley, T.: Current status of anabolic steroids. *JAMA, 184*:527-32, 1963.

189. Fujioka, H., and others: On the anti-fatigue effects of potassium and magnesium salts of 1-aspartic acid as evaluated by several fatigue indexes. *Nat Def Med J, 10*:72-8, 1963.

190. Fujioka, H., and others: Inhibitory effects of 1-aspartic acid salts against fatigue resulting from march. *Nat Def Med J, 10*:525-8, 1963.

191. Fukui, T., and others: The effect of potassium and magnesium aspartates on fatigue. *Tokushima J Exp Med, 9*:24-31, 1962.

192. Furberg, C.: Adrenergic beta-receptor blockade and anaerobic metabolism. *Nature, 211*:888, 1966.

193. Furberg, C.: Adrenergic beta-blockade and physical working capacity. *Acta Med Scand, 182*:119-27, 1967.

194. Furberg, C.: Effects of beta-adrenergic blockade on ECG, physical working capacity and central circulation with special reference to autonomic imbalance. *Acta Med Scand Suppl, 488*:1-46, 1968.

195. Furberg, C., and Ringqvist, T.: Penicillin and working capacity. *Lancet, 1*:622, 1967.

196. Furberg, C., and Schmalensee, G.: Beta-adrenergic blockade and central circulation during exercise in sitting position in healthy subjects. *Acta Physiol Scand, 73*:435-46, 1968.

197. Ganslen, R., and others: Effects of some tranquilizing, analeptic and vasodilating drugs on physical work capacity and orthostatic tolerance. *Aerospace Med, 35*:630-33, 1964.

198. Ganslen, R.: Doping and athletic performance. In Falls, H. (Ed.): *Exercise Physiology.* New York, Acad Pr, 1968.

199. Ganz, V.: The acute effect of alcohol on the circulation and on the oxygen metabolism of the heart. *Am Heart J, 66*:494, 1963.

200. Garlind, T., and others: Effect of ethanol on circulatory, metabolic, and neurohumoral function during muscular work in man. *Acta Pharmacol et Toxicol, 17*:106-14, 1960.

201. Georgescu, M., and others: Dereglarea hipertona in conditii de suprasolicitare fizica si psihica. *Stud Cercet Med Intern, 3*:515-23, 1962.

202. Gilbert, B.: Drugs in sport. *Sports Illustrated, 30*:64-72, June 23, 1969.

203. Gilbert, B.: Something extra on the ball. *Sports Illustrated, 30*:30-42, June 30, 1969.

204. Gilbert, B.: High time to make some rules. *Sports Illustrated, 31*: 30-35, July 7, 1969.
205. Girdano, D., and Girdano, D.: *Drugs—A Factual Account.* Reading, Addison-Wesley, 1973.
206. Goldbarg, A.: *The effects of pharmacologic agents on human performance.* Paper presented at Seminar on Physiology and Psychology of Exercise Testing and Training of Coronary Disease Patients and Coronary Prone Subjects, Airlie, Virginia, April 20, 1972.
207. Goldbarg, A., and others: Therapy of angina pectoris with propranolol and long-acting nitrates. *Circulation, 40*:847-53, 1969.
208. Goldbarg, A., and others: Effects of cigarette smoking on hemodynamics at rest and during exercise. Normal subjects. *Chest, 60*:531-36, 1971.
209. Golding, L.: Drugs and hormones. In Morgan, W. (Ed.): *Ergogenic Aids and Muscular Performance.* New York, Acad Pr, 1972.
210. Golding, L., and Barnard, J.: The effect of d-amphetamine sulfate on physical performance. *J Sport Med, 3*:221-4, 1963.
211. Goldstein, A., and others: Psychotropic effects of caffeine in man. *J Pharm Exp Ther, 149*:156-59, 1965.
212. Goldstein, A., and others: Psychotropic effects of caffeine in man. *J Pharm Exp Ther, 150*:146-51, 1965.
213. Gould, L.: Cardiac effects of alcohol. *Am Heart J, 79*:422-25, 1970.
214. Graf, K., and Strom, G.: Effect of ethanol ingestion on arm blood flow in healthy young men at rest and during work. *Acta Pharmacol et Toxicol, 17*:115-20, 1960.
215. Graf, O.: Zur Frage der spezifischen Wirkung der Cola auf die korperliche Leistungsfahigkeit. *Arbeitsphysiologie, 10*:376-95, 1939.
216. Graham, G., and Bos, R.: *The effect of dextro-amphetamine sulfate on integrated action potentials and local muscular fatigue.* Paper presented at AAHPER National Convention, Houston, Texas, 1972.
217. Grandjean, E., and Abelin, T.: Effect of nicotine on the swimming achievement and atheromatosis of cholesterol-fed rats. *Schweiz Z Sportmed, 12*:132-44, 1964.
218. Gregg, D., and Wiggers, C.: The circulatory effects of acute experimental hypervolemia. *Am J Physiol, 104*:423-32, 1933.
219. Grollman, A.: The action of alcohol, caffeine and tobacco on the cardiac output of normal man. *J Pharmacol, 39*:313, 1930.
220. Gullbring, B., and others: The effect of blood volume variations on the pulse ratio in supine and upright positions and during exercise. *Acta Physiol Scand, 50*:62-71, 1960.
221. Guyton, A.: *Medical Physiology.* Philadelphia, Saunders, 1971.
222. Guyton, A., and Richardson, T.: Effect of hematocrit on venous return. *Circ Res, 9*:157-64, 1961.

223. Haggard, H., and Jellinek, E.: *Alcohol Explored.* Garden City, Doubleday and Doran, 1942.

224. Hahn, F.: Analeptics. *Pharmacol Rev, 12*:447-530, 1960.

225. Haight, J., and others: Human temperature regulation after severe exercise and ethanol. *J Physiol, 208*:22P-23P, 1970.

226. Haldi, J., and Wynn, W.: Action of drugs on the efficiency of swimmers. *Res Quart, 17*:96-101, 1946.

227. Hamer, J., and Sowton, E.: Effects of propranolol on exercise tolerance in angina pectoris. *Am J Cardiol, 18*:354-60, 1966.

228. Hanley, D.: Chairman, Committee for Medical Services, United States Olympic Committee. Personal communication, April 5, 1972.

229. Hanna, J.: The effects of coca chewing on exercise in Quechua of Peru. *Human Biol, 42*:1-11, 1970.

230. Hanna, J.: Further studies on the effects of coca chewing on exercise. *Human Biol, 43*:200-9, 1971.

231. Hanna, J.: Responses of Quechua Indians to coca ingestion during cold exposure. *Am J Phys Anthropol, 34*:273-78, 1971.

232. Hansma, J.: *Drugs and athletics.* Speech presented to Division of Men's Athletics, AAHPER National Convention, Houston, Texas, 1972.

233. Hardinge, M., and others: The effect of forced exercise on body temperature and amphetamine toxicity. *J Pharmacol Exp Ther, 145*:47-51, 1964.

234. Hartley, L., and Saltin, B.: Reduction of stroke volume and increase in heart rate after a previous heavier submaximal work load. *Scand J Clin Lab Invest, 22*:217-33, 1968.

235. Hawk, P.: A study of the physiological and psychological reactions of the human organism to coffee drinking. *Am J Physiol, 90*:380-81, 1929.

236. Hebbelinck, M.: The effects of a moderate dose of alcohol on a series of functions of physical performance in man. *Arch Internat Pharmacod, 120*:402-5, 1959.

237. Hebbelinck, M.: The effect of a moderate dose of ethyl alcohol on human respiratory gas exchange during rest and muscular exercise. *Arch Internat Pharmacod, 126*:214-18, 1960.

238. Hebbelinck, M.: *Spierarbeid en Ethylalkohol.* Brussel, Arsica Uitgaven, 1961.

239. Hebbelinck, M.: The effects of a small dose of ethyl alcohol on certain basic components of human physical performance. The effect of cardiac rate during muscular work. *Arch Internat Pharmacod, 140*:61-67, 1962.

240. Hebbelinck, M.: The effects of a small dose of ethyl alcohol on certain basic components of human physical performance. *Arch Internat Pharmacod, 143*:247-57, 1963.

241. Heimann, H., and others: Experimental psychological differentiation of the effect of 2 psychostimulants (F-1983 and amphetamine) in humans. *Psychopharmacologia, 8*:79-80, 1965.

242. Henry, F., and Fitzhenry, J.: Oxygen metabolism of moderate exercise, with some observations on the effects of tobacco smoking. *J Appl Physiol, 2*:464-8, 1950.

243. Herbst, R., and Schellenberg, P.: Cocain und muskelarbeit. *Arbeitsphysiologie, 4*:203-16, 1931.

244. Herxheimer, H.: Zur Wirkung des Koffeins auf die sportliche Leistung. *Moenchen Med Wochenschr, 69*:1339, 1922.

245. Hettinger, T.: Der Einfluss des Testosterons auf Muskulatur und Kreislauf. *Medizinische Mitteilungen, 21*:140-49, 1960.

246. Hettinger, T.: *Physiology of Strength*. Springfield, Thomas, 1961.

247. Hickman, C.: *Health for College Students*. Englewood Cliffs, Prentice-Hall, 1958.

248. Himwich, H.: The physiology of alcohol. *JAMA, 163*:545-49, 1957.

249. Hoeschen, R., and others: Haemodynamic effects of angina pectoris, and of nitroglycerin in normal and anginal subjects. *Br Heart J, 28*:221-30, 1966.

250. Holliday, A.: A comparison of benzquinamide with pentobarbital and a placebo in regard to effects on performance of a simple mental task by fatigued humans. *Proc West Pharmacol Soc, 7*:75-8, 1964.

251. Holliday, A., and Devery, W.: Effects of drugs on the performance of a task by fatigued subjects. *Clin Pharmacol Ther, 3*:5-15, 1962.

252. Holliday, A., and others: Compound 841F 1983 compared with d-amphetamine and placebo in regard to effects on human performance. *Psychopharmacologia, 6*:192-200, 1964.

253. Hollingworth, H.: The influence of caffeine on mental and motor efficiency. *Arch Psychol, 3*:1-166, 1912.

254. Hollmann, W.: Symposium des Deutschen Sportarztebundes zum Thema Doping. *Sportarzt Sportmed, 2*:45-84, 1966.

255. Hollmann, W., and Venrath, H.: Die Beeinflussung von Herzgrosse, maximaler O_2 Aufnahme und Ausdauergrenze durch ein Ausdauertraining mittlerer und hoher Intensitat. *Der Sportarzt, 14*: 189, 1963.

256. Hollmann, W., and others: Investigations on the effect of digitalis on the strength of human skeletal muscles. *Munchen Med Wochenschr, 107*:1338-40, 1965.

257. Horse Doping: Pharmacology and the Punter. *Nature, 222*:111, 1969.

258. Horst, K., and others: The effect of caffeine, coffee, and decaffeinated coffee upon blood pressure, pulse rate and certain motor reactions of normal young men. *J Pharmacol Exp Ther, 52*:307-21, 1934.

259. Hoyer, I., and Van Zwieten, P.: The central hypotensive action of amphetamine, ephedrine, phentermine, chlorphentermine, and fenfluramine. *J Pharm Pharmacol, 24*:452-8, 1972.

260. Hoyman, H.: Health ethics and relevant issues. *J School Health, 42*:516-25, 1972.

261. Hueting, J., and Poulus, A.: Amphetamine, performance, effort and fatigue. *Pflugers Arch, 318*:260, 1970.

262. Huisking, C.: *Herbs to Hormones.* Essex, Pequot, 1968.

263. Huizinga, J.: *Homo Ludens: A Study of the Play Element in Culture.* Boston, Beacon Pr, 1950.

264. Ikai, M., and Steinhaus, A.: Some factors modifying the expression of human strength. *J Appl Physiol, 16*:157-61, 1961.

265. Imhof, P.: Anabolic steroids and sports. *Schweiz Z Sportmed, 18*:79-85, 1970.

266. International Amateur Athletic Federation. Anti-doping regulations. 1972.

267. Irwin, T.: High school sports flunk the saliva test. *Today's Health, 48*:44-64, October, 1970.

268. Ivy, J.: *The effect of amphetamine on reaction, movement and completion time in relation to time intervals and dosage levels.* Unpublished abstract, University of Maryland, College Park, 1971.

269. Jacob, J., and Michaud, G.: The effect of various pharmacological agents (amphetamine, cocaine, caffeine, hexobarbital, meprobamate, morphine, dextromoramide, 1-methadone, pethidine and CT 3570) on the time of exhaustion and behavior of animals swimming at 20° C. *Med Exp, 2*:323-8, 1960.

270. Jacob, J., and Michaud, G.: Actions of various pharmacologic agents on the exhaustion time and behavior of mice swimming at 20° C. I. Description of the technic actions of amphetamine, cocaine, caffeine, hexobarbital and meprobamate. *Arch Int Pharmacodyn, 133*:101-15, 1961.

271. Jacob, J., and Michaud, G.: Actions of various pharmacological agents on the exhaustion time and behavior of mice swimming at 20° C. II. Analgesics (morphine, dextromoramide, methadone, pethidine and 3570 CT). Influence of repetition of the test. *Arch Int Pharmacodyn, 135*:462-71, 1962.

272. Jacobson, E., and Bass, D.: Effects of sodium salicylate on physiological responses to work in heat. *J Appl Physiol, 19*:33-6, 1964.

273. Jellinek, E.: Effect of small amounts of alcohol on psychological functions. In *Alcohol, Science and Society.* New Haven, *Q J Stud Alcohol,* 1954.

274. Johnson, L., and O'Shea, J.: Anabolic steroids: effects on strength development. *Science, 164*:957-59, 1969.

275. Johnson, L., and O'Shea, J.: The effects of anabolic steroids on blood chemistry profile, oxygen uptake and strength. *Nutr Rep Int, 1*:65-74, 1970.

276. Johnson, L., and others: Anabolic steroid: effects on strength, body weight, oxygen uptake, and spermatogenesis upon mature males. *Med Sci Sports, 4*:43, 1972.

277. Johnson, W., and Black, D.: Comparison of effects of certain blood alkalinizers and glucose upon competitive endurance performance. *J Appl Physiol, 5*:577-78, 1953.

278. Johnson, W., and Jones, J.: Hemodynamic and oxygen transport responses to exercise in hypertensive and normotensive age peers; effects of hypotensive drug treatments. *Am J Med Sci, 253*:180-93, 1967.

279. Jokl, E.: Notes on Doping. In Jokl, E., and Jokl, P. (Eds.): *Exercise and Altitude.* Basel, S. Karger, 1968.

280. Jones, K., and others: *Drugs and Alcohol.* New York, Harper and Row, 1969.

281. Jouglard, J.: Psychotonics and doping. *Arch Mal Prof, 30*:54-6, 1969.

282. Juchems, R.: Hemodynamic effects of ethyl alcohol in man. *Am Heart J, 78*:133-35, 1969.

283. Jurna, I., and others: The action of adrenaline on the fatigued cat soleus muscle. *Experientia, 20*:278-9, 1964.

284. Kahler, R., and others: The effects of autonomic nervous system inhibition on the circulatory response to muscular exercise. *J Clin Invest, 41*:1981-7, 1962.

285. Kalent, J.: A review of physiological and biological studies with alcohol. *Q J Stud Alcohol, 23*:52-93, 1962.

286. Kalent, H., and others: The effect of ethanol on the metabolic rate of rats. *Can J Biochem, 41*:2197-2203, 1963.

287. Kaplan, H., and others: Chloral hydrate and alcohol metabolism in human subjects. *J Forensic Sci, 12*:295-304, 1967.

288. Karpovich, P.: Effect of amphetamine sulfate on athletic performance. *JAMA, 170*:558-61, 1959.

289. Karpovich, P., and Hale, C.: Tobacco smoking and athletic performance. *J Appl Physiol, 3*:616-21, 1951.

290. Karpovich, P., and Millman, N.: Athletes as blood donors. *Res Quart, 13*:166-68, 1942.

291. Karpovich, P., and Sinning, W.: *Physiology of Muscular Activity.* Philadelphia, Saunders, 1971.

292. Karvinin, M., and others: Physical performance during hangover. *Q J Stud Alcohol, 23*:208-15, 1962.

293. Kay, H., and Birren, J.: Swimming speed of the albino rat. II. Fatigue, practice and drug effects on age and sex differences. *J Geront. 13*:378-85, 1958.

294. Kay, H., and Karpovich, P.: Effect of smoking upon recuperation from local muscular fatigue. *Res Quart, 20*:250-56, 1949.

295. Keck, E., and others: Effects of catecholamines and atropine on cardiovascular response to exercise in the dog. *Circ Res, 9*:566-70, 1961.

296. Kerr, A., and Kirklin, J.: Effect of rapid increase of blood volume on atrial pressures and pulmonary blood volume. *Ann Surg, 172*:278-83, 1970.

297. Kinnard, W.: The use of drugs in athletics. *Md State Med J, 19*:67-8, 1970.

298. Klafs, C., and Lyon, M.: *The Female Athlete.* St. Louis, Mosby, 1973.

299. Klausen, K., and others: Effect of high altitude on maximal working capacity. *J Appl Physiol, 21*:1191-94, 1966.

300. Kleemeier, L., and Kleemeier, R.: Effects of benzedrine sulfate (amphetamine) on psychomotor performance. *Am J Psychol, 60*:89-100, 1947.

301. Kleinrok, Z., and Swiezynska, M.: The effect of nialamid, pargylin, methylphenidan, amphetamine, carboethoxyphthalazinehydrazine, benzquinamide, and reserpine on the swimming speed of normal and weighted rats. *Acta Physiol Pol, 17*:659-68, 1966.

302. Knauf, H.: The effect of beta-receptor-blocking agents on the blood flow of the working skeletal muscle. *Z Kreislaufforsch, 58*:749-54, 1969.

303. Knoefel, P.: The influence of phenisopropyl amine and phenisopropyl methyl amine on work output. *Fed Proc, 2*:83, 1943.

304. Kolansky, H., and Moore, W.: Effects of marijuana on adolescents and young adults. *JAMA, 216*:486-92, 1971.

305. Kondo, M.: Evaluation of anti-fatigue effects of asparagine preparation in sedentary study. *Nat Def Med J, 10*:269-74, 1963.

306. Kornetsky, C.: Effects of meprobamate, phenobarbital and dextro-amphetamine on reaction time and learning in man. *J Pharmacol Exp Ther, 123*:216-9, 1958.

307. Kornetsky, C., and others: The effects of dextro-amphetamine on behavioral deficits produced by sleep loss in humans. *J Pharmacol Exp Ther, 127*:46-50, 1959.

308. Korobkov, A., and others: Effect of muscular training and tonic substances on non specific resistance and work capacity in rats. *Fiziol Zh SSSR Sechenov, 47*:30-7, 1961.

309. Kourounakis, P.: Pharmacological conditioning for sporting events. *Am J Pharm, 144*:151-8, 1972.

310. Krebs, H., and others: Effect of ethanol on postexercise lactacidemia. *Isr J Med Sci, 5*:959-62, 1969.

311. Krone, R., and others: Effects of cigarette smoking at rest and during exercise. II. Role of venous return. *J Appl Physiol, 32*:745-8, 1972.

312. Krumholz, R., and Ross, J.: Effect of atropine and reserpine on pulmonary diffusing capacity during exercise in man. *J Appl Physiol, 19*:465-8, 1964.

313. Kruse, C.: Treatment of fatigue with aspartic acid salts. *Northwest Med, 60*:597-603, 1961.

314. Laborit, H., and others: Influence de la composition ionique du mileau extra-cellulaire et influence comparee de l'acid aspartique, de l'aspartate de potassium et du glucose sur l'epreuve de nage du rat blanc. *Compt Rend Soc Biol, 151*:1383-86, 1957.

315. Laborit, H., and others: La place de certains sels de l'acide dl-aspartique dans les mechanismes de conservation de l'activite reactionnelle a l'environment. *Presse Med, 66*:1307-9, 1958.

316. Larson, P., and others: Some effects of nicotine and smoking on metabolic functions. *Clin Pharmacol Ther, 2*:80-109, 1961.

317. Latz, A., and others: Swimming performance of mice as affected by antidepressant drugs and baseline levels. *Psychopharmacologia, 10*:67-88, 1966.

318. Leake, C.: *The Amphetamines: Their Actions and Uses.* Springfield, Thomas, 1958.

319. Leake, C., and Silverman, M.: *Alcoholic Beverages in Clinical Medicine.* Chicago, Year Book Medical, 1966.

320. LeBlanc, J.: Effect of chlorpromazine on swimming time of rats at different temperatures. *Proc Soc Exp Biol Med, 98*:648-50, 1958.

321. Lees, H.: Farewell to benzedrine benders. *Colliers, 124*:32, 1949.

322. Lehman, G., and others: Pervitan als Leistungssteigerndes mittel. *Arbeitsphysiologie, 10*:680-91, 1939.

323. Leon, D., and others: Hemodynamic effects of practolol at rest and during exercise. *Circulation, 45*:46-54, 1972.

324. Leukel, F.: *Introduction to Physiological Psychology.* St. Louis, Mosby, 1968.

325. Levi, L.: The effect of coffee on the function of the sympatho-adrenomedullary system in man. *Acta Med Scand, 181*:431-38, 1967.

326. Levitt, R., and Webb, W.: Effect of aspartic acid salts on exhaustion produced by sleep deprivation. *J Pharm Sci, 53*:1125-6, 1964.

327. Levy, R.: Effects of smoking cigarettes on the heart. *JAMA, 135*: 417-22, 1947.

328. Lieber, C., and Davidson, C.: Some metabolic effects of ethyl alcohol. *Am J Med, 33*:319-27, 1962.

329. Liesen, H., and others: Studies on the influence of propranolol and propranolol with beta-acetyl-digoxin on cardiopulmonary and metabolic parameters during measured work. *Verh Deutsch Ges Kreislaufforsch, 37*:180-6, 1971.

330. Lombard, W.: Some of the influences which affect the power of voluntary muscular contractions. *J Physiol, 13*:1-58, 1892.

331. Lovingood, B.: Effects of d-amphetamine sulfate, caffeine and high temperature on human performance. *Res Quart, 38*:64-71, 1967.

332. Lovingood, B.: Drugs: Effect on human performance. In Larson, L. (Ed.): *Encyclopedia of Sport Sciences and Medicine.* New York, MacMillan, 1971.

333. Lovingood, B., and others: Effects of amphetamine (dexedrine) and caffeine on subjects exposed to heat and exercise stress. *Res Quart, 31*:553-59, 1960.

334. Luebs, E., and others: Effect of nitroglycerin, intensain, isoptin, and papaverine on coronary blood flow in man. *Am J Cardiol, 17*:535-41, 1966.

335. MacDonald, H., and others: Effect of intravenous propranolol on the systemic circulatory response to sustained handgrip. *Am J Cardiol, 18*:333-44, 1966.

336. Machata, G.: The chemical detection of doping among athletes. *Deutsch Z Ges Gerichtl Med, 57*:335-41, 1966.

337. Maglio, A., and others: Research on fatigue prevention (action of 4-hydroxy-19-nortestosterone-17-cyclopentylpropionate). *Ann Med Nav, 68*:797-802, 1963.

338. Maitra, S., and others: Effect of tea drinking on muscular efficiency with special reference to the relief of physiological fatigue. *J Exp Med Sci, 11*:56-62, 1967.

339. Maksud, M., and others: Effects of propranolol on several physiological responses during orthostatic and exercise stress in healthy male subjects. *Can J Physiol Pharmacol, 49*:867-72, 1971.

340. Maksud, M., and others: The effects of physical conditioning and propranolol on physical work capacity. *Med Sci Sports, 4*:225-29, 1972.

341. Margaria, R., and others: The effect of some drugs on the maximal capacity of athletic performance in man. *Int Z Angew Physiol, 20*:281-7, 1964.

342. Margaria, R., and others: Effect of alkalosis on performance and lactate formation in supramaximal exercise. *Int Z Angew Physiol, 29*:215-23, 1971.

343. Marijuana. *Am J Psychiatry, 128*:189-219, 1971.

344. Marozzi, E.: Testing of the Vidic reaction, used for detection of doping in athletes, on several substances of various types. *Farmaco, 19*:173-88, 1964.

345. Marquis, D., and others: Experimental studies of behavioral effects of meprobamate on normal subjects. *Ann NY Acad Sci, 67*:701, 1957.

346. Marshall, R., and others: Effects of epinephrine on cardiovascular and metabolic responses to leg exercise in man. *J Appl Physiol, 18*:1118-22, 1963.

347. Martin, W.: Physiologic, subjective and behavioral effects of amphetamine. *Clin Pharmacol Ther, 12*:245-58, 1971.

348. Martindale, W.: *The Extra Pharmacopoeia.* London, Pharmaceutical, 1972.
349. Matoush, L., and others: Effects of aspartic acid salts (Mg+K) on the swimming performance of rats and dogs. *J Appl Physiol, 19*:262-64, 1964.
350. Maurer, D., and Vogel, V.: *Narcotics and Narcotic Addiction.* Springfield, Thomas, 1967.
351. Mazess, R., and others: Effects of alcohol and altitude on man during rest and work. *Aerospace Med, 39*:403-6, 1968.
352. McIntosh, P.: *Sport in Society.* London, C. A. Watts, 1963.
353. Meck, W., and Eyster, J.: The effect of plethora and variations in venous pressure on diastolic size and output of the heart. *Am J Physiol, 61*:186, 1922.
354. Medical Commission of the British Commonwealth Games: Prevention and detection of drug taking (doping) at the IX British Commonwealth Games. *Scott Med J, 16*:364-8, 1971.
355. Meier, G., and Schumann, R.: Orciprenaline and theophylline effect on the circulatory system during ergometer stress. *Med Klin, 64*:689-92, 1969.
356. Miles, H.: *Alcohol and Human Efficiency.* Washington, Carnegie Institute, 1924.
357. Missiuro, W., and others: Effects of adrenal cortical gland in rest and work. *Am J Physiol, 121*:549-54, 1938.
358. Moerman, E., and de Vleeschhouwer, G.: Detection of doping: separation and identification of amphetamine and related compounds in urine. *Arch Belg Med Soc, 25*:455-61, 1967.
359. Mollet, R.: Current tendencies of modern training. *Am Corr Ther J, 22*:103-11, 1968.
360. Morgan, W.: *Ergogenic Aids and Muscular Performance.* New York, Acad Pr, 1972.
361. Mowar, S.: Anabolic steroids—their uses and side effects. *Indian Med J, 60*:165-8, 1966.
362. Muller, H., and others: Arbeitsversuche mit und ohne Digitalis zur Objectivierung einer latenten Herinsuffizienz bei psychiatrishen Patienten im alter von 50 bis 70 Jahren und Vergleich mit gesunded Kontrollpersonnen zwischen 20 bis 30 Jahren. *Z Kreislaufforsch, 59*:821-43, 1970.
363. Murphy, J., and Eagan, C.: Effects of exercise and anabolic steroids on body and organ weights of mature rats. *Nutr Rep Int, 4*:65-76, 1971.
364. Murphy, R.: The use and abuse of drugs in athletics. *Ohio State Med J, 67*:737-41, 1971.
365. Murray, J., and others: Systemic oxygen transport in induced normovolemic anemia and polycythemia. *Am J Physiol, 203*:720-24, 1962.

366. Murray, J., and others: The circulatory effects of hematocrit variations in normovolemic and hypervolemic dogs. *J Clin Invest,* 42:1150-59, 1963.

367. Musser, R., and O'Neill, J.: *Pharmacology and Therapeutics.* London, MacMillan, 1969.

368. Mustala, O.: Doping. *Duodecim, 80:*132-8, 1964.

369. Mustala, O.: Improvement of athletic performance by drugs. *Suom Laak, 22:*690-5, 1967.

370. Nadel, J., and Comroe, J.: Acute effects of inhalation of cigarette smoke on airway conductance. *J Appl Physiol, 16:*713, 1961.

371. Nagle, F., and others: The mitigation of physical fatigue with Spartase. *Fed Aviat Agency Rep,* 63-12, 10 July 1963.

372. Nair, C., and others: Effect of furosemide (Lasix) on physical work capacity of altitude-acclimatised subjects at an altitude of 11,000 feet. *Aerosp Med, 42:*268-70, 1971.

373. National Collegiate Athletic Association: *The Coach: Drugs, Ergogenic Aids and the Athlete.* Kansas City, Missouri, NCAA, 1971.

374. Naughton, J., and others: Characterization of heart rate response to graded exercise before and after vasodilators. *Med Sci Sports,* 4:33-36, 1972

375. Nazar, K., and others: Mechanism of impaired capacity for prolonged muscular work following beta-adrenergic blockade in dogs. *Pflugers Arch, 336:*72-8, 1972.

376. NCAA testing faces snarls; drug testimony conflicting. *Evening Star,* Washington, June 19, 1973.

377. Nelson, D.: Effects of ethyl alcohol on the performance of selected gross motor tests. *Res Quart, 30:*312-20, 1959.

378. Nicholas, W., and others: Prophylactic use of succinylsulfathiazole and performance capacities. A pilot study of college runners. *JAMA, 205:*757-61, 1968.

379. Nordenfelt, I., and Persson, S.: Haemodynamic effects of propranolol and nitroglycerin in normal subjects during submaximal exercise. *Acta Med Scand, 186:*407-10, 1969.

380. Nordstrom-Ohrberg, G.: Effect of digitalis glucosides on electrocardiogram and exercise test in healthy subjects. *Acta Med Scand Suppl, 420:*1-75, 1964.

381. Ogata, M., and others: Effect of K, Mg-aspartate on fatigue. *J Sci Labour, 38:*705-9, 1962.

382. Oscai, L., and others: Effect of exercise on blood volume. *J Appl Physiol, 24:*622-24, 1968.

383. O'Shea, J.: Anabolic steroids: Effects on competitive swimmers. *Nutr Rep Int, 1:*337-42, 1970.

384. O'Shea, J.: The effects of an anabolic steroid on dynamic strength levels of weightlifters. *Nutr Rep Int, 4:*363-70, 1971.

385. O'Shea, J., and Winkler, W.: Biochemical and physical effects of an anabolic steroid in competitive swimmers and weightlifters. *Nutr Rep Int, 2:*351-62, 1970.

386. Osness, W.: *A study of the effects of dextra amphetamine sulfate on the human organism during exercise.* Paper presented at the AAHPER National Convention, Boston, 1969.

387. Ostyn, M.: Doping among sportsmen. *Psychiatr Neurol Neurochir, 75:*231-4, 1972.

388. Ostyn, M., and Styns, H.: The influence of a blood donation on the work capacity of athletes. *Arch Belg Med Soc, 17:*375-87, 1959.

389. Otsuka, S.: Effect of K, Mg-aspartate administration on fatigue. *J Sci Labour, 40:*229-31, 1964.

390. Pace, N., and others: The increase in hypoxia tolerance of normal man accompanying the polycythemia induced by transfusion of erythrocytes. *Am J Physiol, 148:*152-63, 1947.

391. Palarea, E.: Some physiological effects of alcohol and their application in modern therapeutics. *J Am Geriatr Soc, 11:*933-44, 1963.

392. Palecek, F.: Effects of an anabolic steroid on fatigue and compliance of denervated gastrocnemius. *Acta Endocrinol, 46:*331-35, 1964.

393. Parker, J., and others: The effect of nitroglycerin on coronary blood flow and the hemodynamic response to exercise in coronary artery disease. *Am J Cardiol, 27:*59-65, 1971.

394. Parry, H.: Use of psychotropic drugs by United States adults. *Public Health Reports, 83:*799-810, 1968.

395. Partridge, G.: Studies in the physiology of alcohol. *Am J Psychol, 11:*318-76, 1899.

396. Paul, O., and others: A longitudinal study of coronary heart disease. *Circulation, 28:*20, 1963.

397. Pawan, G.: Physical exercise and alcohol metabolism in man. *Nature, 218:*966-7, 1968.

398. Pawlucki, A.: Doping in sport. *Wiad Lek, 25:*1433-7, 1972.

399. Perman, E.: The effect of ethyl alcohol on the secretions from the adrenal medulla in man. *Acta Physiol Scand, 44:*241-47, 1958.

400. Pierson, W.: Amphetamine sulfate and performance. A critique. *JAMA, 177:*345-47, 1961.

401. Pihkanen, T.: Neurological and physiological studies on distilled and brewed beverages. *Ann Med Exper Biol Fenn, 35:*Suppl 9, 1-152, 1957.

402. Pirnay, F., and others: Influence of amphetamine on some muscular exercise carried on by normal individuals. *Int Z Angew Physiol, 25:*121-9, 1968.

403. Platt, J.: The scientific urgencies of the next ten years. *Rehovot,* Winter, 1969/1970.

404. Pleasants, F., and Grugan, J.: Effects of short periods of abstinence from cigarette smoking on swimming endurance of chronic smokers. *Res Quart, 38*:474-79, 1967.

405. Pleasants, F.: Pretraining and post-training swimming endurance of smokers and nonsmokers. *Res Quart, 40*:779-82, 1969.

406. Policreti, C., and others: Observations on the influence of various psychotropic substances on the attentive capacity of a homogenous group of oarsmen. *Ann Med Nav, 68*:803-8, 1963.

407. Pomeranz, D., and Krasner, L.: Effect of a placebo on a simple motor response. *Percept Motor Skills, 28*:15-8, 1969.

408. Porritt, A.: Doping. *J Sport Med, 5*:166-8, 1965.

409. Potenza, P., and others: On the anti-fatigue action of an oral anabolic drug. *Ann Med Nav, 68*:628-38, 1963.

410. Prichard, B., and Gillam, P.: Assessment of propranolol in angina pectoris. *Br Heart J, 33*:473-80, 1971.

411. Prokop, L.: Adrenals and sport. *J Sport Med, 3*:115-21, 1963.

412. Prokop, L.: The problem of doping. Final report on the international doping conference. FIMS congress, Tokyo, October, 1964. *J Sport Med, 5*:88-90, 1965.

413. Prokop, L.: The struggle against doping and its history. *J Sports Med, 10*:45-8, 1970.

414. Rachman, S.: Effects of stimulant drug on extent of motor responses. *Percept Motor Skills, 12*:186, 1961.

415. Rasch, P., and others: The effect of amphetamine sulfate and meprobamate on reaction time and movement time. *Int Z Angew Physiol, 18*:280-84, 1960.

416. Ray, O.: *Drugs, Society and Human Behavior.* St. Louis, Mosby, 1972.

417. Reeves, W., and Morehouse, L.: The acute effect of smoking upon the physical performance of habitual smokers. *Res Quart, 21*:245-48, 1950.

418. Regatky, E., and others: Effects of guanethidine and propranolol on cardiac adaptation to sinuosoidal exercise. *Rev Soc Argent Biol, 46*:23-9, 1971.

419. Reitan, R.: The comparative effects of placebo, ultran, and meprobamate on psychologic test performance. *Antibiot Med Clin Ther, 4*:158, 1957.

420. Remberg, G., and others: Amphetamine—a metabolite of AN 1. *Arch Toxikol, 29*:153-7, 1972.

421. Replogle, R., and Merrill, E.: Experimental polycythemia and hemodilution: physiological and rheologic effects. *J Thorac Cardiovas Surgery, 60*:582-88, 1970.

422. Richardson, J., and Bassett, W.: Comparison of an anabolic steroid (Dianabol) with a non-steroid weight gaining drug (Periactin) on the effectiveness of muscle building, strength and weight gain in African green monkeys. Research in progress, Old Dominion University, Norfolk, 1973.

423. Richardson, T., and Guyton, A.: Effects of polycythemia and anemia on cardiac output and other circulatory factors. *Am J Physiol, 197*:1167-70, 1959.

424. Richmond Times Dispatch, B 11, February 28, 1973.

425. Riff, D., and others: Acute hemodynamic effects of ethanol on normal human volunteers. *Am Heart J, 78*:592-97. 1969.

426. Rispe, R., and Lucas, H.: Contribution to the study of the effects of salts of aspartic acid on fatigue in combat swimmers. *Bull Soc Med Milit Franc, 54*:158-62, 1960.

427. Rivers, W.: *The Influence of Alcohol and Other Drugs on Fatigue.* London, Edward Arnold, 1908.

428. Rivers, W., and Webber, H.: The action of caffeine on the capacity for muscular work. *J Physiol, 36*:33-47, 1907.

429. Robinson, B., and others: Circulatory effects of acute expansion of blood volume. *Circ Res, 19*:26-32, 1966.

430. Robinson, S., and Harmon, P.: The lactic acid mechanism and certain properties of the blood in relation to training. *Am J Physiol, 32*:757-69, 1941.

431. Rode, A., and Shephard, R.: The influence of cigarette smoking upon the oxygen cost of breathing in near-maximal exercise. *Med Sci Sports, 3*:51-5, 1971.

432. Rodman, T., and others: The effect of digitalis on the cardiac output of the normal heart at rest and during exercise. *Ann Intern Med, 55*:620, 1961.

433. Rokosz, R.: *The effect of d-amphetamine sulfate on the swimming performance of rats.* Unpublished master's thesis, University of Maryland, College Park, 1971.

434. Roney, J. ,and Nall, M.: *Medication Practices in a Community: An Exploratory Study.* Mendo Park, Stanford Research Institute, 1966.

435. Root, W., and Hoffmann, F. (Eds.): *Physiological Pharmacology. I. The Nervous System—Part A.* New York, Acad Pr, 1963.

436. Root, W., and Hoffmann, F. (Eds.): *Physiological Pharmacology. II. The Nervous System—Part B.* New York, Acad Pr, 1965.

437. Rosen, H., and others: Effects of the potassuim and magnesium salts of aspartic acid on metabolic exhaustion. *J Pharm Sci, 51*:592-3, 1962.

438. Roubicek, J.: Doping from the viewpoint of neuropsychiatry. *Cesk Psychiat, 59*:361-6. 1963.

439. Rowell, L., and others: Limitations to prediction of maximal oxygen uptake. *J Appl Physiol, 19*:919-27, 1964.

440. Rudel, R.: Striated muscle fibers: facilitation of contraction at short lengths by caffeine. *Science, 172*:387-88, 1971.

441. Russell, R., and Reeves, T.: The effect of digoxin in normal man on the cardiorespiratory response to severe effort. *Am Heart J, 66*: 381-8, 1963.

442. Ryan, A.: Use of amphetamines in athletics. *JAMA, 170*:562, 1959.

443. Ryde, D.: Sports medicine—the athletes nerves. *J R Coll Gen Pract, 21*:161-3, 1971.

444. Saarne, A., and others: Studies on the nitrogen balance in the human being during long term treatment with different anabolic agents under strictly standardized conditions. *Acta Med Scand, 177*: 199-211, 1965.

445. Saltin, B., and others: Response to submaximal and maximal exercise after bed rest and training. *Circulation, 38*:Supplement 7, 1968.

446. Samuels, L., and others: Influence of methyl-testosterone on muscular work and creatine metabolism in normal young men. *J Clin Endocrinol, 2*:649-54, 1942.

447. Saratikov, A., and others: Effect of pyridrol on energy metabolism in the brain during prolonged muscular activity. *Biull Eksp Biol Med, 72*:35-7, 1971.

448. Schilpp, R.: A mathematical description of the heart rate curve of response to exercise, with some observations on the effects of smoking. *Res Quart, 22*:439-45, 1951.

449. Schroder, G.: Autonomic blocking drugs on circulatory adaptation at rest and during exercise in man; pronethalol and poldine in long term treatment. *Acta Med Scand, 184*:347-52, 1968.

450. Schroeder, G., and others: Hemodynamics during rest and exercise before and after prolonged digitalization in normal subjects. *Clin Pharmacol Ther, 3*:425-31, 1962.

451. Schubert, B.: Identification and metabolism of some doping substances in horses. *Acta Vet Scand Suppl, 21*:1-101, 1967.

452. Schuler, H.: Animal experiments on the problem of body functional power after the intake of caffeine. *Med Klin, 61*:512-3, 1966.

453. Sealey, B., and others: Acute effects of oral alprenolol on exercise tolerance in patients with angina. *Br Heart J, 33*:481-88, 1971.

454. Seashore, R., and Ivy, A.: Effects of analeptic drugs in relieving fatigue. *Psychol Monographs, 67*:1-16, 1953.

455. Segel, N., and Bishop, J.: The circulatory effects of pronethalol with special reference to changes in heart rate and stroke volume during exercise. *Clin Sci, 29*:363-73, 1965.

456. Segers, M., and others: *Le Doping: Traveux du Service d'Etudes de l'INEPS.* Brussels, Institut National de l'Education Physique et des Sports, 1962.

457. Seligson, D., and others: Some metabolic effects of ethanol on humans. *Clin Res Proc, 1*:86, 1953.
458. Seltzer, A., and others: Effect of digoxin on the circulation in normal men. *Br Heart J, 21*:335, 1959.
459. Sex of athletes. *Br Med J, 1*:185-86, 1967.
460. Shah, L., and others: Clinical trials of norcamphane hydrochloride in fatigue states. II. A double blind comparison with d-amphetamine sulfate. *Indian J Med Sci, 21*:645-7, 1967.
461. Shaptala, V., and others: A comparative study of the effect of tea, a fermented grain beverage and black coffee on the functional status of the organism of deep shaft miners. *Vop Pitan, 27*:40-44, 1968.
462. Sharman, I.: Drugs in sport. *Br Med J, 2*:346-7, 1972.
463. Shaw, D., and others: Management of fatigue: a physiologic approach. *Am J Med Sci, 243*:758-69, 1962.
464. Shaw, J.: *Use and misuse of drugs among college athletes.* Paper presented at the American School Health Convention, Chicago, October. 1971.
465. Shephard, R.: *Frontiers of Fitness.* Springfield, Thomas, 1971.
466. Shephard, R.: *Alive Man: The Physiology of Physical Activity.* Springfield, Thomas, 1972.
467. Sidell, F., and Pless, J.: Ethyl alcohol: blood levels and performance decrements after oral administration to man. *Psychopharmacologia, 19*:246-61, 1971.
468. Silva, A., and Leitao, J.: Investigation of the action of glucose, of ATP and of caffeine on fatigue in the rat. *Med Contemp, 79*:311-42, 1961.
469. Silverman M., and others: Effect of isoprenaline on the cardiac and respiratory responses to exercise. *Clin Sci, 42*:13P, 1972.
470. Silvestrini, B.: On doping. *Boll Chimicofarm, 103*:541-4, 1964.
471. Silvette, H., and others: The actions of nicotine on central nervous system function. *Pharmacol Rev, 14*:137-73, 1962.
472. Simonson, E., and Ballard, G.: The effect of small doses of alcohol on the central nervous system. *Am J Clin Pathol, 14*:333-41, 1944.
473. Simonson, E., and others: Effect of oral administration of methyltestosterone on fatigue in eunuchoids and castrates. *Endocrinol, 28*:506-12, 1941.
474. Simonson, E., and others: Effect of methyl testosterone treatment on muscular performance and the central nervous system of older men. *J Clin Endocrinol, 4*:528-34, 1944.
475. Singh, S.: Effects of stimulant and depressant drugs on physical performance. *Percept Motor Skills, 14*:270, 1962.
476. S'Jongers, J., and others: Les effects du doping amphetamique sur la frequence cardiaque, en altitude moyenne simulee en caisson de decompression. *Schweiz Z Sportmed, 17*:21-33, 1969.

477. Sjostrand, T.: *Clinical Physiology.* Stockholm, Svenska Bokforlaget, 1967.

478. Smetzer, D., and others: Cardiovascular effects of amphetamines in the horse. *Can J Comp Med, 36*:185-94, 1972.

479. Smith, G., and Beecher, H.: Amphetamine sulfate and athletic performance. I. objective effects. *JAMA, 170*:542-57, 1959.

480. Smith, G., and Beecher, H.: Amphetamine, secobarbital, and athletic performance. II. subjective evaluations of performance, mood states, and physical states. *JAMA, 172*:1502-14, 1960.

481. Smith, G., and Beecher, H.: Amphetamine, secobarbital and athletic performance. III. quantitative effects of judgment. *JAMA, 172:* 1623-29, 1960.

482. Smith, G., and others: Increased sensitivity of measurement of drug effects in expert swimmers. *J Pharmacol Exp Ther, 139*:114-19, 1963.

483. Smith, J.: An administrator's view of the use and misuse of drugs among athletes. *J School Health, 42*:170-1, 1972.

484. Smith, L., and Dugal, L.: Influence of testosterone on the spontaneous running activity of white rats. *Can J Physiol Pharmacol, 44*:682-86, 1966.

485. Smulyan, H., and others: Effect of beta-adrenergic blockade on the initial hemodynamic response to exercise. *J Lab Clin Med, 71:* 378-89, 1968.

486. Sollman, T.: *Manual of Pharmacology.* Philadelphia, Saunders, 1956.

487. Sommer, S., and Hotovy, R.: The influence of 2-ethylamino-3-phenylnorcamphane on the muscular performance in rats. *Arzneimittelforsch, 12*:472-74, 1962.

488. Sommerville, W.: The effect of benzedrine on mental and physical fatigue in soldiers. *Can Med Assoc J, 55*:470-76, 1946.

489. Sowton, E., and others: Effect of practolol on exercise tolerance in patients with angina pectoris. *Am J Med, 51*:63-70, 1971.

490. Starr, I., and others: A clinical study of the action of ten commonly used drugs on cardiac output, work and size, on respiration, on metabolic rate and on the electrocardiogram. *J Clin Invest, 16*:799-823, 1937.

491. Steinbach, M.: Peculiarities in competitive athletics specific of the group. *Bibl Psychiat Neurol, 142*:121-31, 1969.

492. Stewart, G.: Drugs, performance and responses to exercise in the racehorse. Observations on amphetamine, promazine and thiamine. *Aust Vet J, 48*:544-47, 1972.

493. Stone, E.: Swim-stress-induced inactivity: relation to body temperature and brain norepinephrine, and effects of d-amphetamine. *Psychosom Med, 32*:51-9, 1970.

494. Stone, I.: *The Passions of the Mind.* Garden City, Doubleday, 1971.

495. Swerdlow, M.: General analgesics used in pain relief: pharmacology. *Br J Anaesth, 39*:699-712, 1967.

496. Symposium on beta-adrenergic receptor blockade. *Am J Cardiol,* *18*:303-487, 1966.
497. Talland, G., and Quarton, G.: Effects of drugs and familiarity on performance in continuous visual search. *J Nerv Ment Dis,* *143*:266-74, 1966.
498. Tang, P., and Rosenstein, R.: Influence of alcohol and dramamine, alone and in combination, on psychomotor performance. *Aerospace Med, 38*:818-21, 1967.
499. Tatarelli, G., and others: Pharmacobiological potentiation of the athlete. *Ann Med Nav, 66*:74-81, 1961.
500. Taylor, S., and others: The effect of adrenergic blockade on the circulatory response to exercise in man. *Clin Sci, 28*:117-24, 1965.
501. Terauds, J.: *Physiological effects of methandrostenolone without training.* Paper presented at the AAHPER National Convention, Houston, March, 1972.
502. Theil, D., and Essing, B.: Cocain und Muskelarbeit. I. Der Einfluss auf Leistung und Gasstoffwechsel. *Arbeitsphysiologie, 3*:287-97, 1930.
503. Thomas, C.: *The effects of variant cardiac stress on the peripheral eosinophil count.* Unpublished master's thesis, Old Dominion University, Norfolk, 1972.
504. Thoren, C.: Effects of beta-adrenergic blockage on heart rate and blood lactate in children during maximal and submaximal exercise. *Acta Paediat Scand Suppl, 177*:123-25, 1967.
505. Thorgersen, H., and Lienert, G.: The effect of meprobamate on intellectual test performance with and without stress. *J Psychol, 51*:405-9, 1961.
506. Thornton, G., and others: The effects of benzedrine and caffeine upon performance in certain psychomotor tasks. *J Abnorm Soc Psychol, 34*:96-113, 1939.
507. Toffler, A.: *Future Shock.* New York, Bantam, 1970.
508. Torsti, P., and others: Influence of reserpine, guanethidine and hydrochlorothiazide on tissue catecholamines and metabolism in exercised rats. *Ann Med Exp Biol Fenn, 46*:53-6, 1968.
509. Trancioveanu, M., and others: On the action of neostigmine in the recovery processes in athletes. *Fiziol Norm Patol, 17*:261-8, 1971.
510. Trounce, J.: *Drugs in current use.* New York, Putnam, 1970.
511. Tyler, D.: The effect of amphetamine sulfate and some barbiturates on the fatigue produced by prolonged wakefulness. *Am J Physiol, 150*:253-62, 1947.
512. Ulmark, R.: The dangers of doping. *J Sport Med, 3*:248-9, 1963.
513. Ulrych, M., and others: Immediate hemodynamic effects of beta adrenergic blockade with propranolol in normotensive and hypertensive man. *Circulation, 37*:411-16, 1968.
514. Uyeno, E.: Hallucinogenic compounds and swimming response. *J Pharmacol Exp Ther, 159*:216-21, 1968.

515. Uyeno, E.: Relative potency of amphetamine derivatives and n,n-dimethyltryptamines. *Psychopharmacologia, 19*:381-7, 1971.

516. Van Rossum, J.: Mode of action of psychomotor stimulant drugs. *Int Rev Neurobiol, 12*:307-83, 1970.

517. Vanek, M., and Cratty, B.: *Psychology and the Superior Athlete.* London, MacMillan, 1970.

518. Venerando, A.: Doping: pathology and ways to control it. *Medicina Dello Sport, 3*:972-83, 1963.

519. Venerando, A., and others: Action of amphetamine on the cardiac rate at rest, during muscular work and restoration. *Boll Soc Ital Biol Sper, 42*:164-7. 1966.

520. Venerando, A., and others: Action of amphetamine on muscular work in man. II. Observations on oxygen consumption. *Boll Soc Ital Biol Sper, 42*:613-6, 1966.

521. Venerando, A., and others: Action of amphetamine on muscular work in man. III. Observations of elimination of CO_2. *Boll Soc Ital Biol Sper, 42*:617-19, 1966.

522. Venerando, A., and others: Action of amphetamine on muscular work in man. IV. Observations on respiratory quotient. *Boll Soc Ital Biol Sper, 42*:619-22, 1966.

523. Venerando, A., and others: Action of amphetamine on muscular work efficiency in man. V. Observations on the ventilatory equivalent. *Boll Soc Ital Biol Sper, 43*:454-7, 1967.

524. Venerando, A., and others: Action of amphetamine on muscular work efficiency in man. VI. Observations on the pulse oxygen index. *Boll Soc Ital Biol Sper, 43*:457-60, 1967.

525. Venerando. A., and others: Classification and methods for the detection of some doping agents. *J Sports Med, 9*:245-52, 1969.

526. Vial, C.: *A Contribution to the Study of Neuromuscular Fatigue and its Treatment in Athletics.* Paris, Imprimerie des Tournelles, 1959.

527. Vida, J.: *Androgens and Anabolic Agents.* New York, Acad Pr, 1969.

528. Vidacek, S.: The effect of sympathomimetics on work efficiency under physical effort. *Arh Hig Rada, 16*:136-60, 1965.

529. Villa, R., and Panceri, P.: Action of some drugs on performance time in mice. *Farmaco Prat, 28*:43-8, 1973.

530. Wallace, P.: Auto racing. In Larson, L. (Ed.): *Encyclopedia of Sport Sciences and Medicine.* New York, Macmillan, 1971.

531. Walters, P., and others: Drug use and life-style among 500 college undergraduates. *Arch Gen Psychiat, 26*:92-96, 1972.

532. Walther, H.: On the effect of caffeine and theophylline on the fatigued rat diaphragm preparation. *Arch Int Pharmacodyn, 138*:597-612, 1962.

533. Weiss, B.: Enhancement of performance by amphetamine-like drugs. In Sjoqvist, F., and Tottie, M. (Eds.): *Abuse of Central Stimulants.* Stockholm, Almqvist and Wiksell, 1969.

534. Weiss, B., and Laties, V.: Enhancement of human performance by caffeine and the amphetamines. *Pharmacol Rev, 14*:1-36, 1962.

535. Weiss, U., and Muller, H.: Zur Frage der Beeinflussung des Krafttrainings durch Anabole Hormone. *Schweiz Z Sportmed, 16*:79-89, 1968.

536. Weisse, A., and others: Hemodynamic effects of normovolemic polycythemia in dogs at rest and during exercise. *Am J Physiol, 207*:1361-66, 1964.

537. Wendt, V., and others: Acute effects of alcohol on the human myocardium. *Am J Cardiol, 17*:804-12, 1966.

538. Wenzel, D., and Rutledge, C.: Effects of centrally acting drugs on human motor and psychomotor performance. *J Pharm Sci, 51*: 631-44, 1962.

539. Whitney, A., and Ryan, A.: The effect of acetylsalicylic acid on free fatty acids in blood and possible relationship to aerobic performance. *J Sports Med Phys Fitness, 11*:93-97, 1971.

540. Willgoose, C.: Tobacco smoking, strength, and muscular endurance. *Res Quart, 18*:219-25, 1947.

541. Williams, M., and others: Hemodynamic effects of cardiac glycosides on normal human subjects during rest and exercise. *J Appl Physiol, 13*:417-21, 1958.

542. Williams, M. H.: Effect of selected doses of alcohol on fatigue parameters of the forearm flexor muscles. *Res Quart, 40*:832-40, 1969.

543. Williams, M. H.: Comparison of the submaximal cardiovascular step test response to a maximal aerobic performance task. *Am Correct Ther J, 24*:127-29, 1970.

544. Williams, M. H.: *Relationship of the resting heart rate to submaximal cardiovascular step test performance in athletes and non-athletes.* Paper presented at VAHPER State Convention, Hampton, Virginia, December, 1971.

545. Williams, M. H.: Effect of small and moderate doses of alcohol on exercise heart rate and oxygen consumption. *Res Quart, 43*:94-104, 1972.

546. Williams, M. H.: Effect of plasma, RBC and whole blood transfusion upon oxygen pulse during submaximal work. *VAHPER Res J, 1*:12-14, 1972.

547. Williams, M. H.: The effect of a moderate dose of alcohol on maximal heart rate and maximal endurance capacity. Unpublished data, Old Dominion University, Norfolk, 1972.

548. Williams, M. H., and Thompson, J.: The effect of variant dosages of amphetamine upon performance. *Research Quarterly, 44*:417-22, 1973.

549. Williams, M. H., and others: Effect of blood reinjection upon endurance capacity and heart rate. *Med Sci Sports, 5*:181-86, 1973.

550. Winter, C., and Flataker, L.: Work performance of trained rats as affected by corticoadrenal steroids and by adrenalectomy. *Am J Physiol, 199*:863-6. 1960.

551. Witham, A., and others: The effect of the intravenous administration of dextran on cardiac output and other circulatory dynamics. *J Clin Invest, 30*:897-902, 1951.

552. Wolf, S.: Psychosomatic aspects of competitive sports. *J Sport Med, 3*:157-63, 1963.

553. Wydra, O.: Influence of an anabolic steroid (Dianabol) and muscular training on skeletal muscles of the mouse. *Z Anat Entwicklungsgesch, 136*:73-86, 1972.

554. Wyndham, C., and others: Physiological effects of the amphetamines during exercise. *South African Med J, 45*:247-52, 1971.

555. Yamada, M., and others: Effects of aspartic acid preparate in labor fatigue. *Advances Obstet Gynec, 16*:15-19, 1964.

556. Yu, P., and others: Cardiorespiratory responses and electrocardiographic changes during exercise before and after intravenous digoxin in normal subjects. *Am J Med Sci, 224*:146-53, 1952.

557. Zalis, E., and Parmley, L.: Fatal amphetamine poisoning. *Arch Intern Med, 112*:822-26, 1963.

GLOSSARY

AAU—Amateur Athletic Union

Abolon—Trademark for a preparation of nandrolone decanoate, an anabolic steroid

Acetylsalicylic acid—Aspirin, a pain reliever

Adrenal medulla—The internal aspect of the adrenal gland which secretes the hormones epinephrine and norepinephrine

Adrenalin—Trademark for preparations of epinephrine

Adroyd—Trademark for a preparation of oxymetholone, an anabolic steroid

Aerobic—As related to exercise, the ability to meet energy needs by adequate intake of oxygen

Aerobic power—Synonymous with aerobic capacity or maximal oxygen uptake

Alcohol—C_2H_5OH, a colorless liquid with depressant effects; ethyl alcohol or ethanol

Alkaline reserve—The buffering capacity of the blood

Alkaline salts—Buffering salts such as sodium bicarbonate used to counteract acidity in various parts of the body

Alpha adrenergic receptors—Theoretical substance located in different sympathetic effector organs which responds to only norepinephrine

Amiphenazole—A CNS stimulant, primarily used as a respiratory stimulant

Amobarbital—A white crystalline powder used as a sedative and hypnotic

Amphetamine—Synthetic racemic desoxynorephedrine; a synthetic CNS stimulant

Amphetamine sulfate—A white odorless crystalline power used as a CNS stimulant

Amyl nitrite—A clear yellow liquid, $C_5H_{11}NO_2$, used to relax smooth muscles, causing vasodilation.

Anabolic steroids—Chemical compounds similar to testosterone that facilitate the building of muscular tissue through nitrogen retention; the androgenic effects are minimized

Anaerobic—As related to exercise, the ability to meet energy needs

169

via pathways not requiring immediate sources of oxygen, e.g. glycolysis

Anaerobic capacity—The ability of an individual to rely on anaerobic energy sources; may be used synonymously with oxygen debt capacity

Analgesics—Pain relieving agents without loss of consciousness

Anapolon—Trademark for a preparation of oxymetholone, an anabolic steroid

Anavar—Trademark for a preparation of oxandrolone, an anabolic steroid

Androgens—Substances that produce masculine characteristics such as androsterone and testosterone

Androsterone—An androgen found in the urine of both males and females

Anesthetic—Referring to drugs or agents that are used to abolish the sensation of pain

ANOVA—Analysis of variance; a statistical technique used to test significant differences among mean values

Anti-depressants—Agents that stimulate the mood of depressed individuals

Antihypertensive agents—Agents that counteract high blood pressure

ARAS—Ascending reticular activating system

ASA—Acetylsalicylic acid

Ascending reticular activating system—An intricate system of interlacing nerve cells originating in the spinal cord and extending to the diencephalon; stimulation produces a state of wakefulness in the cerebral cortex

Aspartates—Salts of aspartic acid

Aspartic acid—Asparaginic acid; a hydrolysis product of asparagine, a nonessential amino acid

Astrand-Rhyming test—A submaximal exercise test which attempts to predict maximal oxygen uptake from heart rate response to a standardized workload

ATP—Adenosine triphosphate; the immediate source of energy for muscular contraction

Autogenic technique—Also known as psychotonic training, or the specialized training of an athlete in self-motivation techniques in order to reach high levels of activation for competition

BAL—Blood alcohol level; the concentration of alcohol in the blood

Barbiturates—A drug group used as sedatives or hypnotics

Bemegride—A CNS stimulant primarily affecting the respiratory system

Bennies—Slang for Benzedrine, an amphetamine

Benzedrine—Trademark for a preparation of amphetamine

Benzphetamine—One of the psychomotor and sympathomimetic agents

Berserkers—Legendary Norse warriors who were believed to be invulnerable in battle

Beta adrenergic blocking agents—Drugs or agents that block the stimulation of beta adrenergic receptors in the sympathetic effector organs

Beta adrenergic receptors—Theoretical receptor substance that exists in the various sympathetic effector organs and responds to epinephrine

Bicycle ergometer—A device utilized to administer standardized exercise workloads

Blood doping—A technique aimed at expanding the normal blood volume by infusion of whole blood or packed RBC's

Bradykinin—A kinin composed of a chain of nine amino acids which has been hypothesized to be involved in the etiology of pain

Breathalyzer—An instrument for the detection of blood alcohol levels through breath analysis

Bufotein—Bufotenine; a hallucinogenic agent

Buphenine—A sympathomimetic agent which acts predominantly on beta-adrenergic receptors, increasing peripheral blood flow to the muscles

Butyrophenones—A class of major tranquilizers

Caffeine—A CNS stimulant derived from coffee, tea, and other common plants

Caffeine citrate—A preparation of equal parts of caffeine and citric acid which is utilized as a CNS stimulant

Caffeine sodium benzoate—A white powder composed of equal parts of caffeine and sodium benzoate which is used primarily as a CNS stimulant

Cardiac output—Amount of blood pumped by the heart per minute; minute volume

Cardiac stimulants—Agents used to increase the efficiency of the heart through increased myocardial contraction

Cardiotonic glycoside—Carbohydrate compound occurring in certain plants, such as digitalis, which has a tonic or stimulating action on the heart

Catecholamines—Compounds exerting sympathomimetic effects, such as epinephrine and norepinephrine

Cerebellum—The part of the brain primarily concerned with muscular coordination

Cerebral cortex—The cerebrum, or main portion of the brain

CFL—Continental Football League

Chlordiazepoxide—A minor tranquilizing agent

Chlorpromazine—A phenothiazine derivative; used as a major tranquilizer

Chlorthiazide—An antihypertensive agent

Cholestatic liver damage—Stoppage or suppression of the flow of bile

Chromatography—A method of chemical analysis whereby different compounds are differentiated due to their absorption velocities through various media

Clonidine—An antihypertensive agent

CNS stimulant—Any drug which elicits a stimulating effect upon the central nervous system

Coca—The leaves of Erythroxylon coca, from which cocaine is derived

Cocaine—A crystalline alkaloid used as a systemic stimulant and local anaesthetic

Compazine—Trademark for a preparation of prochlorperazine; a major tranquilizer of the phenothiazine class

Congener—A substance allied by nature, origin, or function to another

Control conditions—Comparative conditions in experimental designs whereby all variables, except the experimental variables, are controlled so as to have valid comparisons

Criterion measure—In doping experimentation, the exercise task used to evaluate the effect of the drug

D-amphetamine—Dextro-amphetamine; the dextrorotary isomer of amphetamine sulfate; a more powerful amphetamine than the racemic form

Danabol—Trademark for methandrostenolone, an anabolic steroid

Deca-Durabolin—Trademark for a preparation of nandrolone decanoate, an anabolic steroid

Demand characteristics—The subject's alteration in behavior during experimentation, based upon various cues, which may be biased towards substantiating the experimenter's hypothesis

Depressants—Agents that diminish functional activity of the CNS

Desoxyephedrine—Methamphetamine; methylamphetamine; used as a CNS stimulant

Dexedrine—Trademark for d-amphetamine sulfate

Dextromoramide—A narcotic analgesic used in the treatment of moderate to severe pain

Dianabol—Trademark for methandrostenolone, an anabolic steroid

Diencephalon—The thalamus and hypothalamus

Diethylbarbituric acid—A hypnotic and sedative agent

Diethylpropion—A stimulant drug used also as an anoretic ,or appetite suppressant

Digitalis—The dried leaves of Digitalis purpurea; used as a cardiac glycoside, or cardiac stimulant

Diphenylmethane derivatives—A class of tranquilizing agents

Dipipanone—A potent narcotic analgesic

Dipyridamole—An agent used to improve coronary circulation

Diuretic—An agent that increases the secretion of urine

DL-amphetamine—Equimolecular mixture of the dextrorotary and levorotary forms of amphetamine

DMT—Dimethyltryptamine, a hallucinogenic agent

DNA—Deoxyribonucleic acid

DOM—The active hallucinogenic substance of STP

Doping—The use of drugs in athletics in order to achieve a physiological or psychological advantage

Dose response—The fact that the behavioral changes may be dependent upon the amount of the drug administered

Double-blind—An experimental design in which neither the investigator nor the subject has knowledge of the drug treatment used

Durabolin—Trademark for a preparation of nandrolone phenylpropionate, an anabolic steroid

Dynamometer—A mechanical device utilized to measure isometric strength

Ephedrine—A sympathomimetic agent used as a CNS stimulant or to relieve bronchial spasm

Epinephrine—A natural sympathomimetic secreted by the adrenal medulla

Equanil—Trademark for a preparation of meprobamate

Ergogenic aids—Agents which are utilized in attempts to increase work capacity

Ergograph—A recording of work output

Ergometer—A device used to measure work output

Estrogen—A generic term for estrus producing agents

Ethanol—Ethyl alcohol

Ethyl alcohol—The basic alcohol used for human consumption

Ethylamphetamine—One of the psychomotor stimulants

Ethyloestrenol—An anabolic and androgenic agent; proprietary preparations include Orabolin and Maxibolin

Fencamfamin—A CNS and psychomotor stimulant banned by the IAAF; H610

Fenproporex—A psychomotor stimulant banned by the IAAF

FFA—Free fatty acids

FISM—International Federation of Sports Medicine

Fluid retention—Action of certain drugs, such as anabolic steroids, which retain body water.

Gas-liquid chromatography—Chromatography in which the mixture of substances to be separated is vaporized in a stream of carrier gas that moves over a suitably supported stationary liquid phase.

GLC—Gas-liquid chromatography

Glyceryl trinitrate—Nitroglycerin, a vasodilator

Glycogen—The chief storage of carborydrate in the human body, primarily in the liver and muscle

Glycogenolysis—The splitting of glycogen in the tissues

Greenies—Combination of amphetamines and barbiturates used to produce beneficial effects of both stimulation and depression

Hallucinogens—Agents capable of producing distortion of the senses with possible hallucinations

Halo effect—Tendency of an investigator to generalize his feelings to a subject based upon his knowledge of the subject's role in the experiment; may be controlled by double-blind experimentation

Hashish—The stalks and leaves of Cannabis indica; a hallucinogenic compound

Hawthorne effect—The effect on the subject's performance due to knowledge that he is involved in an experiment; may be controlled by placebo designs

Heroin—A narcotic analgesic; diacetylmorphine

Hypervolemia—Increase in blood volume above normal

Hypnosis—An artificially induced condition whereby the individual is increasingly amenable to suggestions

Hypnotics—Agents that induce sleep

Hypoglycemia—Lowered blood sugar levels

Hypothalamus—The part of the diencephalon that controls autonomic activities, water balance, temperature, and other important body activities

IAAF—International Amateur Athletic Federation

Information feedback—Control of information or stimuli administered to a subject during or after experimentation in order to affect his response

Informed consent—Prior knowledge communicated to subjects relative to the nature of the experiment in which they will be involved

In vitro—Within a glass or test tube; outside the human body

In vivo—Within the living body

IOC—International Olympic Committee

Isometric—Muscular contraction without movement; static contraction

Isosorbide dinitrate—A drug used in the treatment of coronary insufficiency

Isotonic—Muscular contraction with movement; dynamic contraction

Khat—Catha leaves, containing norpseudoephedrine, a CNS stimulant

KPM—A measure of work done; kilopound meter or kilogram meter; equals 7.23 foot pounds of work

Lactic acid—The anaerobic end product of glycolysis; it has been implicated as a causative factor in the etiology of fatigue

L-amphetamine—Levorotary amphetamine

Leptazole—A CNS stimulant

Lethal dose—The amount of an agent that causes death

LSD—Lysergic acid diethylamide

Lysergic acid diethylamide—A potent hallucinogenic compound derived from the fungus of Claviceps purpurea

Magnesium aspartate—Magnesium salt of aspartic acid; magnesium aminosuccinate tetrahydrate

Major tranquilizer—Depressants that reduce psychotic symptoms

MAOI agents—Monoamine oxidase inhibitors

Marijuana—The leaves and flowering tops of Cannabis sativa, a hallucinogenic agent

Mass spectroscopy—The technique of deflecting electrified particles into separate streams according to their respective masses and thus identifying elements by their mass spectrum

Maxibolin—Trademark for a preparation of ethyloestrenol, an anabolic agent

Maximal oxygen uptake—The ability of the body to utilize oxygen for energy purposes; reflects the product of cardiac output times arterial-venous oxygen difference

Maximal VO$_2$—Maximal oxygen uptake

Medulla oblongata—The nervous tissue at the base of the brain which is continuous with the spinal cord below and the pons above

Mental practice—Practice of a physical skill through mental contemplation of the factors involved in the execution of that skill

Meprobamate—A minor tranquilizer

Mescaline—Toxic hallucinogenic oil extracted from the peyote plant

Methamphetamine—A potent psychomotor stimulant; methylamphetamine; desoxyephedrine

Methandienone—An anabolic steroid; methandrostenolone

Methandriol—An anabolic agent with actions similar to methandienone

Methandrostenolone—17-alpha-methyltestosterone, used as an anabolic hormone; methandienone

Methedrine—Trademark for a preparation of methamphetamine

Methoxyphenamine—A sympathomimetic agent banned by the IAAF

Methyl dopa—An antihypertensive agent

Methylephedrine—A sympathomimetic amine

Methylphenidate—An agent used as a mild psychomotor stimulant

Metrazol—Trademark for preparations of pentylenetetrazol

Micro-infrared spectroscopy—A technique of identifying substances through measurement of the absorption of energy in the infrared spectrum

Miltown—Trademark for a preparation of meprobamate

Minor tranquilizer—Depressants used primarily for the treatment of anxiety and tension

Minute ventilation—Amount of lung ventilation per minute

Monoamine oxidase inhibition—Inhibition of monoamine oxidases which allows noradrenaline and other catecholamines to accumulate; results in indirect stimulation

Morphine—A potent narcotic analgesic; the principle alkaloid of opium

Nandrolone decanoate—An anabolic agent; deca-Durabolin is one of the proprietary preparations

Nandrolone phenpropionate—An anabolic agent; Durabolin is one of the proprietary preparations

Narcotic—Any agent that produces insensibility to pain

NCAA–National Collegiate Athletic Association

Negatively ionized air–Ionic imbalance in the air that has been theorized to produce a stimulating effect

Neurohormone–A hormone stimulating the neural mechanism

NFL–National Football League

Nicotine–A colorless fluid alkaloid which may be found in tobacco

Nicotinyl tartrate–A vasodilator

Nikethamide–A CNS stimulant affecting primarily the respiratory system

Nilevar–Trademark for a preparation of norethandrolone, an anabolic agent

Nitrogen retention–Increased retention of nitrogen, a basic element in protein, in the muscle tissues as a function of anabolic steroids

Nitroglycerin–Glyceryl trinitrate, a vasodilator

Noradrenaline–Norepinephrine; levarterenol

Norandrostenolone–Nandrolone, an anabolic steroid

Norepinephrine–A hormone secreted by the adrenal medulla with sympathomimetic effects; noradrenaline; levarterenol

Norethandrolone–An anabolic agent similar to methandienone

Normovolemia–Normal blood volume

Norpseudo ephedrine–A CNS stimulant derived from the leaves of Catha edulis; Catha leaves also known as khat

Orabolin–A trademark for a preparation of ethyloestrenol, an anabolic steroid

Oranabol–Trademark for a preparation of oxymesterone, an anabolic steroid

Over-the-counter-drug–Drugs which may be purchased without prescription

Oxanamide–A minor tranquilizer

Oxandrolone–An anabolic steroid

Oxymesterone–An anabolic steroid; Oranabol is one proprietary preparation

Oxymetholone–An anabolic steroid

Pemoline–A psychomotor stimulant with actions between those of amphetamine and caffeine

Perceptual motor–Referring to combined perception of various stimuli and resultant motor response

Periactin–Trademark for preparations of cyproheptadine hydrochloride, used as an antihistamine

Pervitin–Trademark for methamphetamine; desoxyephedrine

Pethidine–A narcotic analgesic

pH–The symbol used to express the alkalinity or acidity of a solution; pH 7 is neutral, above 7 is alkaline and below 7 is acidic

Pharmacology–The study of the action of drugs in all aspects

Phendimetrazine–A psychomotor stimulant similar to amphetamine

Phenelzine–An antidepressant with MAOI action

Phenmetrazine–A psychomotor stimulant and sympathomimetic used primarily as an appetite reducer

Phenobarbital–A hypnotic and sedative agent

Phentermine–A psychomotor stimulant

Phosphocreatine–A high energy compound in the muscle used to regenerate ATP following muscular contraction

Physical working capacity–A general term for physical fitness, usually related to general endurance capacity of the cardiovascular-respiratory type

Pipradol–A psychomotor stimulant and CNS stimulant

Placebo–An inactive substance utilized in experimental studies in order to determine the efficacy of medicaments

Polycythemia–An increase in the number of red corpuscles in the blood

Potassium aspartate–Potassium salt of aspartic acid; potassium amino-succinate hemihydrate

Potassium citrate–The potassium salt of citric acid

Potentiation–The combined action of two drugs, being greater than the sum of the effects of each drug acting separately; synergistic effect

PRE–Progressive resistive exercise

Progesterone–A female hormone whose prime function is to prepare the uterus for the fertilized ovum

Progressive resistive exercise–A training technique, primarily with weights, whereby resistance is increased as the individual develops increased strength levels

Prolintane–A psychomotor stimulant

Promazine–A tranquilizer of the phenothiazine class

Propranolol–A beta-adrenergic blocking agent; antagonizes the actions elicited by beta-adrenergic stimulation

Protein supplementation–Increase in daily dietary protein, usually via high quality protein tablets or powder

Psilocybin–A hallucinogenic compound derived from the mushroom Psilocybe mexicana Heim

Psychedelic–Agents producing freedom from anxiety and eliciting highly enjoyable and creative perceptual changes and thought patterns

Psychodepressants–Agents that reduce the excitability of the CNS and produce sedative or hypnotic effects

Psychomotor–Pertaining to motor effects of cerebral or psychic activity; action of certain drugs to increase motor activity through cerebral stimulation

Psychotogenic–Producing a state of psychosis

Psychotomimetic–Producing symptoms resembling psychoses

Psychoton–A CNS stimulant

Psychotonic–Exerting a stimulating effect on the mind

Psychotoxic–Exerting a poisonous effect on the mind

Psychotropic–A modification of mental activity

Pulmonary diffusing capacity–The capacity of the lungs and pulmonary blood to exchange gases in a given amount of time

PWC–Physical working capacity

PWC$_{170}$–A submaximal work test which predicts maximal work capacity from a submaximal heart rate

Rauwolfia alkaloids–Hypotensive or tranquilizing agents derived from the Rauwolfia genus, particularly the species Rauwolfia serpentina

Reaction time, complex–The voluntary response of an individual to a stimulus, with the response dependent upon a decision-making process

Reaction time, simple–The voluntary response of an individual to a stimulus, usually either visual, auditory, or tactile

Repeated measures design–An experimental design whereby each subject is tested on the criterion measure several times under different treatment conditions

Reserpine–A major tranquilizer derived from Rauwolfia serpentina

Ritalin–Trademark for a preparation of methylphenidate, a stimulant

RNA–Ribonucleic acid

Ronical–Roniacol; nicotinyl alcohol; a peripheral vasodilator

Rosenthal effect–Possible biasing of behavioral studies due to results expected by the experimentor; may be eliminated by double-blind conditions

Secobarbital–One of the barbiturates used as a sedative and hypnotic

Seconal–Trademark for preparations of secobarbital

Sedatives—Agents that reduce excitement or activity of various body functions

SGOT—Serum glutamic oxalacetic transaminase; high levels may indicate heart or liver damage

Sodium bicarbonate—A white, crystalline powder used as an alkalizing agent; $NaHCO_3$, commonly known as baking soda

Sodium citrate—A white crystalline salt used as an alkalizing agent

Sparine—Trademark for preparations of promazine, a tranquilizer

Spartase—Trademark for a preparation of potassium and magnesium aspartates

Stanozolol—A steroid with strong anabolic and weak androgenic properties

Stenediol—Trademark for preparations of methandriol, an anabolic agent

Stimulant—A general agent that produces stimulation; different agents may produce general body stimulation or affect selected parts of the body

STP—A synthetic hallucinogen

Stroke volume—Amount of blood pumped by the heart each beat

Stromba—Trademark for a preparation of stanozolol, an anabolic steroid

Strychnine—A potent CNS stimulant derived from Strychnos nux-vomica

Submaximal exercise—Exercise level below maximal capacity characterized by lower values for heart rate, oxygen uptake, and other physiological responses

Sympathetic nervous system—The branch of the autonomic nervous system that prepares the individual for increased energy demands

Sympathomimetic—Referring to agents which elicit physiological changes normally produced by stimulation of the sympathetic branch of the autonomic nervous system; sympatheticomimetic

Synergistic action—Potentiation

Syrosingopine—An antihypertensive and tranquilizing agent

Testosterone—The male sex hormone produced in the testes which produces and maintains the male secondary sex characteristics

Tetrahydrocannabinol—THC, believed to be responsible for the psychoactive properties of marijuana

Thalamus—The part of the diencephalon which serves as the main relay center for sensory impulses to the cerebral cortex

THAM—Trometamol

Theobromine–An alkaloid used as a smooth muscle relaxant

Theophylline–A white odorless alkaloid derived from tea and used as a smooth muscle relaxant

Thin layer chromatography–Chromatography in which the porous solid is a thin uniform layer of material applied over a glass plate, and separation is achieved by adsorption, partition, or a combination of both processes

Thioxanthenes–A class of major tranquilizers

Thorazine–A trade name for a preparation of chlorpromazine

Time dependent–Indicative of the fact that the action of a drug may be dependent upon various time factors

TLC–Thin layer chromatography

Toxic dose–A drug dosage which will elicit poisonous effects

Tranquilizer–A drug that depresses the CNS, thus relieving anxiety and tension

Trometamol–An organic amine base used to increase the blood pH and treat metabolic or respiratory acidosis

t-test–A statistical test used to determine whether or not a significant difference exists between two means

Vasodilators–Agents which relax the smooth muscles of the vasculature, therefore increasing the caliber of the blood vessels

Vasomotor–Referring to agents which affect the caliber of a blood vessel

Venesection–Withdrawal of blood from a vein by needle insertion

Ventilatory equivalent–The ratio of the amount of lung ventilation necessary to sustain a given oxygen uptake level

Veratrum alkaloids–Derivatives of the Veratrum genus, a lilaceous plant, which are used as tranquilizers

Wheat germ oil–A bland yellow oil with actions and uses of vitamin E

WIN·19,583–A stimulant

Winstrol–Trademark for a preparation of stanozolol

AUTHOR INDEX

Abboud, F., 24
Abelin, T., 57
Aberg, H., 120
Adams, G., 67
Adamson, G., 35, 36, 67, 68, 70, 72
Adolph, J., 78, 80
Ahlborg, B., 102, 105
Albrecht, E., 110, 114
Albrecht, H., 110, 114
Aldinger, E., 122
Alles, G., 35, 53, 54
Anderson, J., 58
Ariel, G., 99, 100
Ariens, E., 15
Asmussen, E., 54, 85, 124
Astrand, P., 102, 113, 117, 119
Astrom, H., 126, 127

Balke, B., 109, 110
Ballard, G., 83
Banister, E., 24
Barbi, G., 126
Bard, P., 111
Barnard, J., 39
Barnard, R., 125
Barnes, R., 103
Bartak, K., 32, 33, 37, 39
Bass, D., 64
Bassett, W., 100
Battig, K., 27, 28, 30, 57
Baugh, R., 7
Beckett, A., 13
Beecher, H., 30, 40, 41, 68, 69, 73, 130, 134
Begbie, G., 77
Berne, R., 111
Birren, J., 27
Bishop, J., 126, 127
Black, D., 118
Blatter, K., 126

Blomqvist, G., 78, 79, 80
Bobo, W., 79, 80
Boje, O., 8, 26, 46, 49, 52, 54, 66, 75, 85, 88, 119, 120, 123, 124
Bollinger, A., 126, 129
Borg, G., 38, 72
Bos, R., 35, 36
Bousvaros, G., 123
Bouton, J., 7
Bowers, R., 95, 98, 101
Brick, I., 126
Broun, H., ix
Brown, B., 92, 95
Brown, C., 58
Brown, H., 94, 97, 101
Bruce, R., 71, 121, 124
Brzezinska, A., 128
Bugyi, G., 54
Bujas, Z., 35, 36, 38, 72
Burch, G., 86
Burger, A., 55
Burn, J., 55
Burt, J., 15
Buterbaugh, G., 67

Caldwell, L., 106
Cameron, J., 30
Campos, F., 24
Carlsson, C., 71
Carpenter, J., 51, 77
Carr, W., 126, 127
Cartoni, G., 13
Casner, S., 94, 97
Catton, B., 7, 52
Cavalli, A., 13
Chaterjee, A., 29
Cheney, R., 51
Chenowith, L., 75
Chidsey, C., 71
Christensson, B., 123

Clarke, E., 11
Clarke, K., 14, 15
Cobley, J., 89
Cochran, W., 43
Cohen, S., 46
Collier, H., 63
Coltart, D., 126
Comroe, J., 56
Consolazio, C., 107
Cooper, D., 5
Cooper, K., 57, 59
Coopersmith, S., 76
Cooter, G., 28
Costello, C., 36, 72
Cox, B., 90
Craig, A., 19
Crancer, A., 60
Cratty, B., 6, 17, 18
Cronin, R., 126, 127
Csaky, T., 6, 130, 135
Cuiffardi, T., 45
Cumming, G., 71, 126, 127
Cuthbertson, D., 31, 37
Cutinelli, L., 102

Dagenais, G., 126
Danysz, A., 35, 41
Danzinger, R., 71
Darling, R., 63, 64
De Crinis, K., 124
De Cristofaro, D., 112
Dennig, H., 117, 118
Detry, J., 124
Devery, W., 31
de Vleeshhouwer, G., 13
de Vries, H., 15, 67, 86, 108, 113, 116, 120
de Wijn, J., 110
Dill, D., 25, 118
Doctor, R., 74, 78
Donald, D., 129
Downey, J., 63, 64

Eagan, C., 92, 95
Eckstein, J., 24
Ekblom, B., 109, 115, 126, 127, 128, 129

Ekstrom-Jodal, B., 127
Epstein, S., 126, 127
Essing, B., 46
Evans, W., 106
Eysenck, H., 31
Eyster, J., 111

Fahey, T., 94, 97, 101
Fallis, N., 105, 106
Feldscher, D., 92, 95
Feigen, G., 35, 53, 54
Ferguson, T., 112
Fewings, J., 79
Finley, S., 35, 36, 67, 68, 70, 72
Fischbach, E., 10, 11, 49, 52, 75
Fisher, A., 63
Fitzhenry, J., 57
Floor-Wieringa, A., 126
Flory, C., 31
Foldi-Borcsok, E., 28
Foltz, E., 38, 53
Forney, R., 77
Foss, M., 125
Fowler, W., 5, 15, 93, 96, 97
Francesconi, A., 135
Frankenhaeuser, M., 69
Frawley, T., 88
Freed, D., 89, 90
Frenkl, R., 90
Frommel, E., 43
Fruehan, A., 88
Fujioka, H., 102, 104, 105
Fukui, T., 104
Furberg, C., 5, 126, 127

Ganslen, R., 54, 71, 72, 124
Ganz, V., 78
Garlind, T., 79, 80, 85
Gilbert, B., 8, 26, 130
Gilbert, J., 31
Gillam, P., 126
Girdano, D., 40, 55, 66
Girdano, D., 40, 55, 66
Goldbarg, A., 57, 126, 127, 129
Golding, L., 39, 102, 108
Goldstein, A., 48
Gould, L., 74, 78, 79

Graf, K., 79, 80, 85
Graham, G., 35, 36
Grandjean, E., 57
Grollman, A., 78
Grugan, J., 58
Gullbring, B., 114
Guyton, A., 55, 91, 96, 112

Haggard, H., 75
Hahn, F., 24
Haldi, J., 41, 54
Hale, C., 58
Hamer, J., 126
Hanley, D., 15
Hanna, J., 46, 47
Hardinge, M., 43
Hartley, L., 78
Hawk, P., 51
Hebbelinck, M., 77, 78, 83, 85
Heimann, H., 31
Henry, F., 57
Herxheimer, H., 53
Hettinger, T., 96
Hickman, C., 75
Hoeschen, R., 123
Hoffman, F., 67
Holliday, A., 31
Hollingsworth, H., 51
Hollman, W., 110, 122
Hotovy, R., 29
Hoyer, I., 32
Hoyman, H., 16
Hueting, J., 32, 34, 39
Huisking, C., 45
Huizinga, J., vii

Ikai, M., 35, 62, 75, 84
Imhof, P., 99, 126
Irwin, T., 7
Ivy, A., 31, 41, 48
Ivy, J., 32

Jacob, J., 28, 46, 50, 65, 68
Jacobson, E., 64
Jellinek, E., 75, 83

Johnson, L., 94, 95, 98, 101
Johnson, W., 118
Jokl, E., 75
Juchems, R., 78
Jurna, I., 25

Kahler, R., 24
Kaplan, H., 78
Karpovich, P., 39, 41, 58, 109, 118
Karvinin, M., 78
Kay, H., 27, 58
Keck, E., 25
Kinnard, W., 9
Klafs, C., 19
Kleemeier, L., 31
Kleemeier, R., 31
Kleinrok, Z., 27, 68
Knauf, H., 127
Knoefel, P., 37
Knox, J., 31, 37
Kondo, M., 104
Kornetsky, C., 31, 69
Kourounakis, P., 10, 15, 48, 49, 55, 62, 135
Krone, R., 57
Krumholz, R., 70
Kruse, C., 104

Laborit, H., 103
Larson, P., 56
Laties, V., 26, 52, 54, 55
Latz, A., 27
Leake, C., 49
Le Blanc, J., 67
Lees, H., 11
Lehman, G., 37
Leukel, F., 55
Levi, L., 48
Levy, M., 111
Levy, R., 57
Liesen, H., 126, 127
Liu, C., 112
Lombard, W., 81
Lovingood, B., 26, 31, 32, 35, 43, 51, 54
Luebs, E., 123
Lyon, M., 19

Maglio, A., 95
Maksud, M., 126, 127, 128
Margaria, R., 32, 33, 39, 54, 119
Marozzi, E., 13
Marshall, R., 25
Martin, W., 30, 32
Martindale, W., 48, 52
Matoush, L., 104
Mazess, R., 78, 80
Meck, W., 111
Merrill, E., 112, 113
Michaud, G., 28, 46, 50, 65, 68
Millman, N., 109
Moerman, E., 13
Mollet, R., 8
Morehouse, L., 58
Morgan, W., 5, 134
Muller, H., 97, 121
Murphy, J., 92, 95
Murphy, R., 14, 66
Murray, J., 112
Mussar, R., 61
Mustala, O., 15, 26, 49, 89
Myrsten, A., 69

Nadel, J., 56
Nagle, F., 106
Naughton, J., 123
Nazar, K., 128
Nelson, D., 77, 83, 85
Nicholas, W., 5
Nordstrom-Ohrberg, G., 121

O'Neill, J., 61
Oscai, L., 110
O'Shea, J., 93, 94, 97, 98, 101
Osness, W., 32, 33, 37
Ostyn, M., 15

Pace, N., 114
Palarea, E., 73
Palecek, F., 92
Panceri, P., 50
Parker, J., 122, 123
Parmley, L., 44
Partridge, G., 82
Paul, O., 50

Pawlucki, A., 14, 15
Perkins, R., 74, 78
Perman, E., 74, 79
Petz, B., 35
Pierson, W., 42, 43
Pihkanen, T., 84
Pilch, A., 92, 95
Pirnay, F., 32, 33, 34
Platt, J., ix
Pleasants, F., 58
Pless, J., 77
Policreti, C., 31, 68
Porritt, A., 11, 15
Poulas, A., 32, 34, 39
Prichard, B., 126
Prokop, L., 12, 15, 136

Quarton, G., 31

Rachman, S., 31
Rasch, P., 25, 31, 70
Ray, O., 3, 45, 48, 55
Reardon, J., 95, 98, 101
Reeves, T., 121
Reeves, W., 58
Regatky, E., 126, 127
Reitan, R., 69
Replogle, R., 112, 113
Richardson, J., 100
Richardson, T., 112
Riff, D., 78, 79
Ringqvist, T., 5
Rivers, W., 53, 81, 82
Robinson, B., 112, 113
Rodahl, K., 102, 113, 117, 119
Rode, A., 56
Rodman, T., 121
Rokosz, R., 28
Root, W., 67
Rosen, H., 103, 106
Rosenstein, R., 77
Ross, J., 70
Roubicek, J., 14
Rowell, L., 109
Rudel, R., 50
Russell, R., 121
Rutledge, C., 31, 51, 70

Ryan, A., 63
Ryde, D., 66

Saarne, A., 93
Saltin, B., 78, 110
Samuels, L., 96
Saville, W., 99
Schilpp, R., 57
Schmalensee, G., 126, 127
Schroeder, G., 121
Schubert, B., 12
Sealey, B., 126
Seashore, R., 31, 41, 48
Segel, N., 126, 127
Segers, M., 26, 32, 33
Selkirk, T., 75
Seltzer, A., 121
Shah, L., 30
Sharman, I., 11
Shaw, D., 104
Shephard, R., 42, 44, 46, 48, 52, 55, 56,
    75, 76, 77, 89, 109
Sidell, F., 77
Silverman, M., 32, 33
Silvette, H., 55
Simonson, E., 83, 96
Singh, S., 36
Sinning, W., 118
S'Jongers, J., 32
Sjostrand, T., 110
Skranc, O., 32, 33, 37, 39
Smith, G., 30, 40, 41, 42, 68, 69, 73,
    130, 134
Smith, J., 7
Sollman, T., 17, 76
Sommer, S., 29
Sommerville, W., 41
Sowton, E., 126
Steinhaus, A., 35, 62, 75, 84
Stewart, G., 29, 68
Stone, I., 45
Strom, G., 79, 80, 85
Swerdlow, M., 62, 64
Swiezynska, M., 27, 68

Talland, G., 31
Tang, P., 77
Tatarelli, G., 7

Theil, D., 46
Thomas, C., 113
Thompson, J., 32, 39
Thoren, C., 125, 126, 129
Thornton, G., 31, 51, 53
Toffler, A., ix, 3
Toohey, J., 90
Trounce, J., 64
Tyler, D., 31

Ulmark, R., 75, 123
Uyeno, E., 27, 60

Van Rossum, J., 24, 46
Van Zwieten, P., 32
Vanek, M., 6, 17, 18
Venerando, A., 8, 12, 26, 32, 33, 49
Venrath, H., 110
Vial, C., 105
Vida, J., 88
Vidacek, S., 44
Villa, R., 50

Wallace, P., 26
Walther, H., 50
Webber, H., 53
Weiss, B., 26, 44, 52, 54, 55
Weiss, U., 97
Weisse, A., 112, 113
Wendt, V., 78
Wenzel, D., 31, 51, 70
Whitney, A., 63
Willgoose, C., 58
Williams, M., 121
Williams, M. H., 32, 39, 78, 79, 80, 84,
    85, 113, 115
Winkler, W., 98, 101
Wolf, S., 75
Wydra, O., 92
Wyndham, C., 34, 37
Wynn, W., 41, 54

Yamada, M., 102
Yu, P., 121

Zalis, E., 44

SUBJECT INDEX

A

AAHPER, 11
AAU, 16, 26, 49
Abolon, 88
Aborigines, Australian, 7
Acetylsalicylic acid (*see* Aspirin)
Adrenalin, 10, 24, 25, 48, 55
Adroyd, 88
Aerobic capacity (*see also* Oxygen
    uptake)
  amphetamine, effects of, 37-39
  caffeine, effects of, 52, 54
  digoxin, effects of, 121
  smoking, effects of, 58, 59
Alcohol, ethyl, 4, 10, 11, 13, 51, 61, 62,
    73-86
  biphasic hypothesis, 74
  effects of chronic ingestion, 86
  effects on
    blood vessels, 79-80
    general endurance, 85, 86
    physiological adjustments to
      exercise, 77-80
      cardiac output, 79
      heart rate, 77-79
      oxygen uptake, 80
      respiratory quotient, 80
      respiratory rate, 80
      ventilatory quotient, 80
    power, 82
    psychomotor performance, 76, 77
    rate of fatigue, 82-84
    reaction time, 77
    running speed, 85
    strength and endurance, 80-86
  metabolism of, 73, 74
  subjective effects, 76
  use in athletics, 74-76
Alkalies (*see* Alkaline salts)

Alkaline salts, 4, 18, 116-119
  and blood pH, 116
  effects on
    anaerobic work capacity, 118, 119
    lactic acid, 119
    oxygen debt, 117-119
    physical working capacity, 117-119
    running performance, 118, 119
    swimming performance, 118
  use in athletics, 116, 117
Amateur Athletic Union (*see* AAU)
American Association of Health,
    Physical Education and
    Recreation (*see* AAHPER)
American College of Sports Medicine,
    25
Amines, sympathomimetic, 9
Amiphenazole, 9, 22
Amobarbital, 38, 72
Amphetamines and similar stimulants,
    4, 10, 14, 18, 22-45, 49, 55
  and temperature regulation during
    exercise, 43, 44
  detection of in humans, 12, 13
  effects on
    aerobic work capacity, 37-39
    anaerobic work capacity, 33, 34
    general endurance, 37-40
    local muscular endurance, 34-36
    physiological adjustments to
      exercise, 32-34
      blood lactate, 32
      blood pressure, 32
      carbon dioxide production, 33
      heart rate, 32
      minute ventilation, 33
      oxygen pulse, 33
      oxygen uptake, 32
      respiratory quotient, 33
      respiratory rate, 32, 33
      ventilatory equivalent, 33

psychomotor performance, 31, 32
  movement time, 31
  reaction time, 31
running performance
  in animals, 29
  in humans, 41, 42
shot putting, 41, 42
strength, 34-36
swimming performance
  in animals, 27-29
  in humans, 41, 42
throwing performance, 41, 42
lethal dose, 44
pharmacological action, 23
subjective effects, 30
use in athletics, 24
Amyl nitrite, 122
Anabolic steroids (*see also* specific
  drugs), 4, 10, 13, 15, 18, 87-102
and female athletes, 89
and protein supplementation, 93-102
and weight training, 93-102
detection of, 90
effects on
  body weight and composition,
    91-95
  oxygen uptake, 101
  reflex time, 99
  strength, 95-102
  strength maintenance, 100
  swimming performance, 101
health hazards, 90
types, 88
use in athletics, 88-91
Anaerobic work capacity (*see also*
  Oxygen debt)
alkalies, effects of, 118, 119
amphetamines, effects of, 33, 34
Analgesia, 61
Analgesics, 13, 61, 62-65
mild, 62-64
narcotic, 10, 64, 65
potent, 64, 65
Anapolon, 88
Anavar, 88
Andean Indians, 7, 46
Androgenic steroids (*see also*
  Anabolic steroids), 87-102

Androstenolone, 96
Antidepressants, 10, 20, 21, 23
ARAS, 21
Archery, 17, 67
ASA (*see* Aspirin)
Ascending reticular activation system
  (*see* ARAS)
Asparaginic acid, 102
Aspartates, 4, 18, 102-108
and fatigue in humans, 104
effects on
  endurance capacity, 103-108
  oxygen debt, 107
  oxygen uptake, 107
  physical working capacity, 103-108
  running performance, 105-107
  strength, 106, 107
  subjective state of mind, 104
  swimming performance in animals,
    103, 104
use in athletics, 102, 103
Aspartic acid, salts of (*see* Aspartates)
Aspirin, 20, 48, 61, 62-64
and exercise in the heat, 64
effects on
  endurance capacity, 63
  FFA mobilization, 63
  heart rate, 63
  maximal running time, 63
  oxygen debt, 63
  oxygen uptake, 63
Athletes
deaths of, due to doping, 14, 43
education of, against doping, 16
female, 18, 19, 89
  and anabolic steroids, 89
subjective state of mind
  amphetamines, effects of, 30
  aspartates, effects of, 104
  secobarbital, effects of, 68, 69
typology of, 17-19
Athletic associations (*see* specific
  organizations)
Athletics
doping, prevalence in, 7, 8
factors contributing to success in,
  17-19
Australian aborigines, 7
Autogenic technique, 6

B

BAL, 74
Barbiturates, 8, 18, 62, 65
Baseball, 18
Bemegride, 9, 22
Bennies, 7
Benzedrine, 8, 11, 27, 41
Benzodiazepine, 66
Benzphetamine, 9, 22
Berserkers, 6
Biological engineering, 3
Biphasic hypothesis, 82
Blood alcohol levels (*see* BAL)
Blood doping, 11, 109-116
  effects on
    physical working capacity, 114-116
    physiological adjustments to
      exercise, 111-116
      cardiac output, 111-113
      heart rate, 112, 113, 116
      oxygen uptake, 112, 113, 115
      oxygen pulse, 113
      oxygen transport, 112, 113
      stroke volume, 112, 113
  physiological effects of, 111-114
  therapeutic effect, 110
  use in athletics, 109-111
Blood flow, muscle
  nitroglycerin, effects of, 124
  propranolol, effects of, 127
Blood infusion (*see* Blood doping)
Blood pressure
  amphetamines, effects of, 32
Body weight and composition
  anabolic steroids, effects of, 91-95
Boxing, 7, 18
Bufotein, 7
Buphenine, 122
Butyrophenones, 66

C

Caffeine, 4, 8, 11, 48-55
  and coronary heart disease, 50
  and endurance bicyclists, 52
  effects on
    aerobic capacity, 54
    endurance capacity, 52-55

high jump performance, 54
isometric strength and endurance,
  50, 52-55
oxygen uptake, 54
physical working capacity, 50-55
psychomotor performance, 51, 52
rate of fatigue, 54
reaction time, 51, 52
running speed, in humans, 54
running performance, in animals,
  50
swimming performance
  in animals, 50
  in humans, 54
use in athletics, 48, 49
Caffeine sodium benzoate, 53
Cannabis sativa, 59
Carbond dioxide production
  amphetamines, effects of, 33
Cardiac glycosides (*see* Digitalis and
  other cardiotonic glycosides)
Cardiac output
  effects of
    alcohol, 79
    blood doping, 111-113
    digitalis, 121
    nitroglycerin, 123
    propranolol, 127
    tranquilizers, 71
Cardiac stimulants (*see* Cardiovascular
  drugs)
Cardiotonic glycosides (*see* Digitalis
  and other cardiotonic glycosides)
Cardiovascular drugs, 4, 10, 13, 18,
  119-129
  digitalis and other glycosides,
    120-122
  nitroglycerin and other vasodilators,
    122-125
  propranolol and other beta-blocking
    agents, 125-129
Cerebellum, 64
Cerebral cortex, 21, 48, 55, 74
CFL, 8
Chlordiazepoxide, 66
Chlorpromazine, 66, 67, 70, 71
Chlorthiazide, 70, 71
Chromatography, 12, 13
  gas liquid, 12

paper, 12
thin layer, 12
Clonidine, 71
CNS stimulants, 9, 10, 20, 21, 22
Coca-Cola, 45
Coca leaves, 7, 45, 47
Cocaine, 8, 9, 21, 22, 45-47
  effects on
    endurance capacity, 46, 47
    physical working capacity, 46, 47
    physiological adjustments to
      exercise
        heart rate, 47
        oxygen uptake, 47
      swimming performance, in animals,
        46
      ventilation, 47
  pharmacological action of, 46
Codeine, 64
Coffee, 7, 48, 49
  reaction time, effect on, 51
Committee on Medical Aspects of
  Sports of AMA, 89
Committee on Sports Medicine of the
  American Academy of Science, 89
Compazine, 66
Continental Football League (*see* CFL)
Council on Drugs of the AMA, 103

D

D-amphetamine (*see also*
  Amphetamines and similar
  stimulants), 27, 28, 30, 31,
  35, 36, 39, 43
Danabol, 88
Deca-Durabolin, 88, 97
Deaths (*see* Athletes, deaths of)
Demand characteristics, 133
Depressants, 17, 61-86
  alcohol, 73-86
  analgesics, 62-65
    mild, 62-64
    potent, 64-65
  sedatives, 65-73
  tranquilizers, 65-73
Desoxyephedrine, 37, 38
Detection methods (*see* Doping,
  detection of)

Dexfenmetrazin, 33, 37, 39
Dextromoramide, 10, 62, 64, 65
Dianabol (*see also* Methandienone),
  88, 90, 92, 94, 95, 97, 98, 100
Diethylbarbituric acid (*see also*
  Veronol), 72
Diethylpropion, 9, 22
Digitalis and other cardiotonic
  glycosides, 12, 119, 120-122
  effects on
    muscular endurance, 121, 122
    physical working capacity, 121
    physiological adjustments to
      exercise, 121, 122
      cardiac output, 121
      heart rate, 121
      lactate production, 121
      oxygen debt, 121
      oxygen transport, 121
      oxygen uptake, 121
      stroke volume, 121
      ventilation, 121
    strength, 122
Digitalis purpurea, 120
Digoxin, 121
  effect on aerobic capacity, 121
Dimethylamphetamine, 9, 22
Dimethylandrostan, 92
Diphenylmethane derivatives, 66
Dipipanone, 10, 62, 64
Dipyridamole, 123
Dl-amphetamine, 28
D-methamphetamine, 30
DMT, 59
DOM, 59
Doping, 6-19
  blood (*see* Blood doping)
  definition, 8-11
  detection, 11-14, 90
    methods, 12, 13
    problems of, 13, 14
  education against, 134-136
  ethics, paradox of, 14-16
  experimental methodology, 132-134
  history of, 6, 7
  in athletics, theoretical values of,
    16-19
  in horses, 11

legislation against, 14-16
medical complications, 14, 90
prevalence in athletics, 7, 8
  college, 7
  high school, 7
  professional, 7, 8
problems in interpreting research,
    130, 131
research considerations, 132-134
research needs, 44, 45, 130-134
Double blind research, 133
Drug revolution, 3
Drug use in athletics (*see* Doping)
Drugs, 3-136
  affecting the cardiovascular system,
    109-129
  affecting the muscular system, 87-108
  affecting the nervous system, 20-86
    depressants, 61-86
    stimulants, 20-60
Durabolin (*see also* Nandrolone
  phenpropionate), 88

E

Education, 134-136
  of athletes against doping, 16,
    134-136
Endurance capacity
  alcohol, effects on, 80-86
  amphetamine, effects on, 34-36
  aspirin, effects on, 63
  aspartates, effects on, 103-108
  caffeine, effects on, 52-55
  cocaine, effects on, 47
  digitalis, effects on, 121, 122
  propranolol, effects on, 127-129
  smoking, effects on, 58, 59
  tranquilizers, effects on, 72
Ephedrine, 9, 10, 11, 22, 23, 30
Epinephrine, 24, 125
Equanil, 66, 67, 71, 72
Ergogenic aids, 4-6
  theory of use, 4
  types, 4
Erythroxylon coca, 46
Esberitox, 28
Ethanol (*see* Alcohol, ethyl)

Ethics, 14-16, 65
Ethyl alcohol (*see* Alcohol, ethyl)
Ethylamphetamine, 9, 22
Ethyloestrenol, 88
Exercise
  tranquilizing effects, 67

F

Female athlete (*see* Athletes, female)
Federation International of Sports
  Medicine (*see* FISM)
Fencamfamin, 9, 22
Fenproporex, 9, 22
Figure ice skating, 18, 67
FISM, 15, 49
Football, 17, 18

G

Glyceryl trinitrite, 122
Golf, 17
Greenies, 7
Gymnastics, 18

H

H610 (*see* Norcamphane
  hydrochloride)
Hallucinogenic drugs, 59, 60
Halo effect, 133
Hashish, 59
Hawthorne effect, 133
Heart rate
  effects of
    alcohol, 77-79
    amphetamine, 32
    aspirin, 63
    blood doping, 112, 113, 116
    cocaine, 47
    digitalis, 121
    nitroglycerin, 123
    propranolol, 126
    smoking, 57
    tranquilizers, 71
Heroin, 10, 12, 64

Hexobarbital, 68
High jumping
    caffeine, effect on, 54
Hormones, 10
    adrenalin (*see* Adrenalin)
    androgenic (*see* Anabolic steroids)
    epinephrine (*see* Epinephrine)
    estrogen, 19
    progesterone, 19
Horses, racing, 11
    amphetamines, effects on, 29
    doping of, 11, 12
    tranquilizers, effects on, 68
Hydrazene derivatives, 23
Hyperthermia
    and amphetamines, 43, 44
    and nikethamide, 43
Hypervolemia, 111-113
Hypnosis, 4, 5, 61
Hypnotics, 61, 65-73
Hypothalamus, 21, 56

I

IAAF, 9, 10, 16, 49, 62, 64, 90
Ice skating, 18, 67
Indians
    Andean, 7, 46
    Quechua, 46
Information feedback, 6
Informed consent, 132
International Amateur Athletic
    Federation (*see* IAAF)
International Cycling Union, 11
International Federation of Sports
    Medicine (*see* FISM)
International Olympic Committee
    (*see* IOC)
IOC, 9, 11, 16, 62, 64, 75, 90
    medical commission of, 10, 21
Isometric strength (*see* Strength)
Isoprenaline, 32
Isosorbide dinitrate, 123
Isosorbide nitrite, 122

L

Lactic acid, 116
    alkaline salts, effects of, 119

amphetamine, effects of, 29, 33, 34
    digitalis, effects upon, 121
Legislation
    against doping, 6
Leptazole, 9, 22
Librium, 66, 68
LSD, 59, 60
    and swimming performance of rats,
        60
Lysergic acid diethylamide (*see* LSD)

M

Magnesium asparates, 102
MAOI agents, 23
Marijuana, 59, 60
Mass spectroscopy, 12, 13
Maxibolin, 88
Maximal oxygen uptake (*see*
    Oxygen uptake)
Medical Commission, British
    Commonwealth Games, 26
Medulla oblongata, 21, 48, 64
Mental practice, 6
Meprobamate, 66-70, 72
Mescaline, 59
Methadone, 10, 62, 64, 65
Methamphetamine, 37, 44
Methandienone (*see also* Dianabol), 88
Methandriol (*see also* Stenediol), 88
Methandrostenolone, 92, 95, 97
Methoxyphenamine, 9, 22
Methylamphetamine, 9, 22, 29, 39
Methyl dopa, 71
Methylephedrine, 9, 22
Methylphenidate, 9, 22, 30
Methyl phenidyl acetate, 32
Methyltestosterone, 96
Metrazol, 41
Micro-infrared spectroscopy, 12, 13
Miltown, 66
Minute ventilation
    amphetamine, effects of, 33
Monoamine oxidase inhibiting agents
    (*see* MAOI agents)
Morphine, 10, 20, 22, 61, 62
    effect on swimming performance in
        animals, 65

Movement time, 18
amphetamines, effect of, 31
Muscular endurance (*see* Endurance capacity)
Muscular strength (*see* Strength)

N

Nandrolone decanoate, 88, 92, 94
Nandrolone phenpropionate (*see also* Durabolin), 88
Narcotic analgesics, 10, 64
National Collegiate Athletic Association (*see* NCAA)
National Federation of State High School Athletic Associations, 9
National Football League (*see* NFL)
NCAA, 7, 9, 13, 16, 49, 90, 131
NFL, 8, 14
Nibal, 93, 97
Nicotine, 22, 55-59
effect on performance in animals, 57
Nicotinic acid, 122
Nicotinyl tartrate, 122
Nike, 7
Nikethamide, 9, 22, 23, 43
Nilevar, 88
Nitroglycerin and other vasodilators, 12, 13, 14, 18, 122-125
effects on
physical working capacity, 124, 125
physiological adjustments to exercise
cardiac output, 123
heart rate, 123
oxygen uptake, 124
muscle blood flow, 124
stroke volume, 123
Norcamphane hydrochloride, 29, 30
Norepinephrine, 23, 24, 46, 70, 125
Norethandrolone, 88
Normovolemic polycythemia (*see* Polycythemia)
Norpseudo ephedrine, 9, 22
Nylidrine hydrochloride, 124

O

Octyl nitrite, 122
Olympics, 5, 7, 8, 14, 49, 54, 66, 75, 110
Orabolin, 88
Oranabol, 88
Oxanamide, 70
Oxandrolone, 88, 93, 96, 98
Oxygen consumption (*see* Oxygen uptake)
Oxygen debt
effects of
alkaline salts, 117-119
aspartates, 107
aspirin, 63
digitalis, 121
propranolol, in dogs, 125
smoking, 57
Oxygen pulse
effects of
amphetamine, 33
blood doping, 113
Oxygen transport
effects of
blood doping, 112
digitalis, 121
Oxygen uptake, 109
effects of
alcohol, 80
amphetamines, 33
anabolic steroids, 101
aspartates, 107
aspirin, 63
blood doping, 112, 113, 115
caffeine, 54
cocaine, 47
digitalis, 121
nitroglycerin, 124
propranolol, 125, 127
smoking, 57
tranquilizers, 71
Oxymesterone, 88
Oxymetholone, 88
Oxypertine, 67, 68, 70, 72

P

Pemoline, 9, 22
Penicillin, 5

Periactin, 100
Peripheral vasodilators (*see also*
    Nitroglycerin and other
    vasodilators), 4
Pervitin (*see also* Desoxyephedrine), 37
Pethidine, 10, 62, 64, 65
Pharmacological potentiation of athletes
    (*see* Doping)
Phenacetin, 63
Phenamine, 38
Phendimetrazine, 9, 22
Phenelzine, 27
Phenmetrazine, 9, 22, 30, 32
Phenobarbital, 66, 69, 70
Phenothiazines, 66
Phentermine, 9, 22
Physical working capacity (*see also*
    Endurance capacity)
  effects of
    alcohol, 85, 86
    anabolic steroids, 95-102
    aspartates, 103-108
    blood doping, 114-116
    caffeine, 52-55
    cocaine, 47
    digitalis, 121, 122
    nitroglycerin, 124, 125
    propranolol, 127-129
    smoking, 58-59
    tranquilizers, 72
Piperazine compounds, 66
Piperioine compounds, 66
Pipradol, 9, 22
Pipradrol hydrochloride, 23
Pituitary gland, 21
Pituri plant, 7
Placebo treatments, 15, 133, 135
Polycythemia, 111-114
Potassium aspartates, 102
Potassium citrate, 116, 118, 119
Power, 18, 82, 83
Prolintane, 9, 22
Promazine, 68
Pronethalol, 128
Propranolol and other beta-blocking
    agents, 125-129
  effects on
    blood flow, muscular, 127

physical working capacity, 126-129
    of cardiac patients, 126
    of children, 125, 126
physiological adjustments to
    exercise
    arteriovenous oxygen difference,
      127
    cardiac output, 127
    heart rate, 126
    oxygen debt, 125
    oxygen uptake, 125, 127
    stroke volume, 127
    running endurance, 129
    running speed, in greyhounds, 129
    subjective state of mind, 129
Psilocyblin, 59
Psychedelic drugs, 59, 60
Psychomotor performance
  effects of
    alcohol, 76, 77
    amphetamines, 31, 32
    caffeine, 51, 52
    tranquilizers, 69, 70
Psychomotor stimulants (*see*
    Amphetamines and similar agents)
Psychotomimetic drugs, 22, 59, 60
Psychotton, 33, 37, 39
PWC (*see* Physical working capacity)

Q

Quechua Indians, 46
Quid, 45

R

Racing
  horses (*see* Horses, racing)
  motor car, 18
Rate of fatigue
  effects of
    alcohol, 82-84
    caffeine, 54
Rauwolfia alkaloids, 66, 67, 71, 122
Reaction time, 18
  effects of

alcohol, 51, 77
amphetamine, 31
caffeine, 51
coffee, 51
tranquilizers, 69, 70
Recordil, 124
Reflex time
effect of anabolic steroids, 99
Reserpine, 66-68, 70, 71
Respiratory quotient
effects of
alcohol, 80
amphetamine, 33
Respiratory rate
effects of
alcohol, 80
amphetamines, 33
Riflery, 17, 67
Ritalin, 38
Ronical, 122
Rosenthal effect, 133
Running endurance
effects of
alkaline salts, 118, 119
amphetamines
in animals, 29
in humans, 39, 41, 42
anabolic steroids, in animals, 95
aspartates, 105-107
aspirin, 63
blood doping, 115, 116
caffeine, in animals, 50
propranolol, 129
tranquilizers, 73
Running speed (*see* Speed)

S

Secobarbital, 30, 68, 73
effects on
running performance, 41, 42, 73
subjective state of mind, 68, 69
swimming performance, 41, 42, 73
throwing performance, 41, 42, 73
Seconal, 72
Sedatives (*see also* specific drugs), 61,
65-73

Self-hypnosis, 6
Shot putting
effects of
amphetamines, 42
secobarbital, 73
Skiing, 18
Smoking, 55-59
effects on
aerobic capacity, 58
muscular endurance, 58
physical working capacity, 58, 59
physiological adjustments, 56, 57
airway conductance, 56
heart rate, 57
lung diffusing capacity, 57
oxygen cost of breathing, 56
oxygen debt, 57
peripheral venous return, 57
stroke volume, 57
power, 58
speed, 58
strength, 58
swimming performance, 58
Sodium citrate, 116, 118, 119
Sodium bicarbonate, 116, 118, 119
Solcoseryl, 114
Spanish conquistadors, 45
Sparine, 66
Spartase, 106
Spectroscopy, 12, 13
mass, 12, 13
micro-infrared, 12, 13
Speed
running
effects of
alcohol, 85
caffeine, 54
propranolol, in dogs, 129
stimulants, in horses, 29
tranquilizers, in horses, 68
swimming
effects of
amphetamine, in anmials, 27, 28
smoking, 58
Sport, universality of, 8
Sports (*see also* specific sports)
typology of, 17-18
Stanozolol, 88, 92, 94, 95, 97

Stenediol, 88
Steranabol, 95
Steroids, anabolic (*see* Anabolic
    steroids)
Stimulants, 18, 20-60, 119-129
    of cardiovascular system, 119-129
    of CNS, 20-60
STP, 59
Strength, 18
    effects of
        alcohol, 80-83
        amphetamines, 34-36
        anabolic steroids, 95-102
        aspartates, 106, 107
        caffeine, 52-55
        digitalis, 122
        smoking, 58
        tranquilizers, 36, 72
Stroke volume
    effects of
        blood doping, 112, 113
        digitalis, 121
        nitroglycerin, 123
        propranolol, 127
        smoking, 57
Stromba, 88
Strychnine, 9, 12, 20, 22
Subjective effects
    of alcohol, 76
    of amphetamines, 30
    of aspartates, 104
    of propranolol, 129
    of secobarbital, 68, 69
    of tranquilizers, 68, 69
Swimming performance
    endurance, animal
        effects of
            amphetamines, 27-29
            anabolic steroids, 95
            aspartates, 103, 104
            caffeine, 50
            cocaine, 46
            morphine, 65
            nicotine, 57
            tranquilizers, 67, 68
    endurance, humans
        effects of
            alkaline salts, 118

amphetamines, 41, 42
        anabolic steroids, 101
        smoking, 58
        tranquilizers, 73
    speed, animals
        effect of LSD, 60
    speed, humans
        effects of
            amphetamines, 41, 42
            anabolic steroids, 101
            caffeine, 54
Sympathetic receptors, 23, 125
Sympathin, 24
Sympathomimetic agents (*see*
        Amphetamines and similar agents)
Syrosingopine, 71

T

Tea, 48, 49
Team sports (*see* specific sport)
Temperature regulation
    amphetamine, effect of during
        exercise, 43, 44
Tennis, 17, 18
Testosterone, 87, 91, 96
Tetrahydrocannabinols, 59
Thalamus, 21
THAM (*see* Trometamol)
Theory
    of drug use in athletics, 5, 16
Thiazole derivatives, 66
Thioxanthenes, 66
Thorazine, 66
Throwing performance
    effects of
        amphetamines, 41, 42
        secobarbital, 73
Tranquilizers (*see also* specific drugs),
        10, 13, 17, 22, 62, 65-73
    effects on
        muscular endurance, 72
        physical working capacity, 71
        physiological adjustments to
            exercise, 70, 71
        cardiac output, 71

heart rate, 71
  oxygen uptake, 71
psychomotor performance, 69, 70
reaction time, 69, 70
running performance, 73
strength, 36, 72
subjective state of mind, 68, 69
swimming performance
  in animals, 67, 68
  in humans, 73
throwing performance, 73
major, 66
minor, 66
sympathomimetic effects, 67
use in athletics, 66, 67
Trometamol, 117
Typology of athletes, 17-19

U

Ultran, 69

V

Vasodilation
  effects of alcohol, 79, 80
Vasodilators (*see* Nitroglycerin and
  other vasodilators)
Ventilation
  effects of
    cocaine, 47
    digitalis, 121
Ventilatory equivalent
  effects of amphetamines, 33
Ventilatory quotient
  effects of alcohol, 80
Veratrum alkaloids, 67
Veronol, 72
Vidic test, 13

W

Weight lifting, 18
  and anabolic steroids, 93-102
Winstrol, 88
WIN•19,583, 35, 36